THE **BIG BOOK** OF

PREGNANCY
NUTRITION

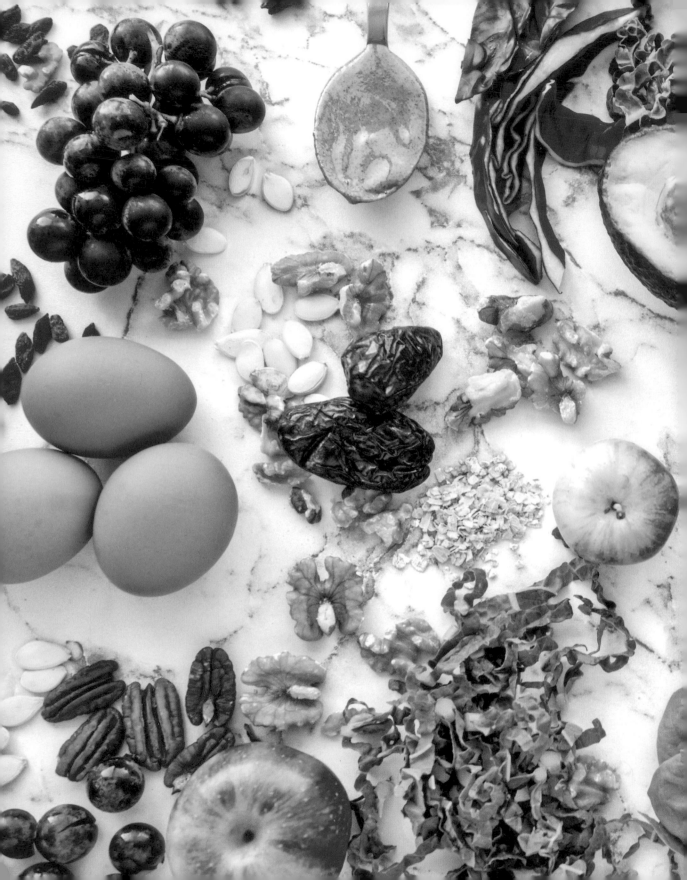

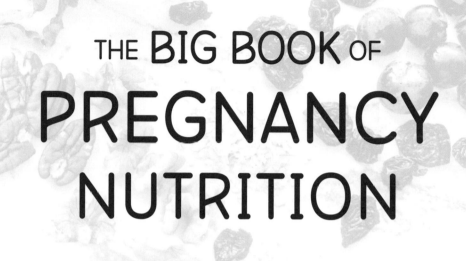

THE BIG BOOK OF PREGNANCY NUTRITION

Everything Expectant Moms Need to Know for a Happy, Healthy Nine Months & Beyond

STEPHANIE MIDDLEBERG
MS, RD, CDN

AVERY | AN IMPRINT OF PENGUIN RANDOM HOUSE | NEW YORK

AVERY

an imprint of Penguin Random House LLC
penguinrandomhouse.com

Photographs © Gabriela Herman

Most Avery books are available at special quantity discounts for bulk purchase for sales promotions, premiums, fundraising, and educational needs. Special books or book excerpts also can be created to fit specific needs. For details, write SpecialMarkets@penguinrandomhouse.com.

Library of Congress Cataloging-in-Publication Data

Names: Middleberg, Stephanie, author.
Title: The big book of pregnancy nutrition: everything expectant moms need to know for a happy, healthy nine months and beyond / Stephanie Middleberg, MS, RD, CDN.
Description: New York: Avery, an imprint of Penguin Random House, [2024] | Includes bibliographical references and index.
Identifiers: LCCN 2023025233 (print) | LCCN 2023025234 (ebook) | ISBN 9780593543450 (trade paperback) | ISBN 9780593543467 (epub)
Subjects: LCSH: Pregnancy—Nutritional aspects—Popular works. | Pregnant women—Health and hygiene—Popular works.
Classification: LCC RG559.M535 2024 (print) | LCC RG559 (ebook) | DDC 618.2—dc23/eng/20230929
LC record available at https://lccn.loc.gov/2023025233
LC ebook record available at https://lccn.loc.gov/2023025234

Printed in China

10 9 8 7 6 5 4 3 2 1

Book design by Lorie Pagnozzi

To Julian and Remi,
you two are the reason this book exists.
Thank you both for bringing me such immense joy
and also for putting up with all the taste testing!

CONTENTS

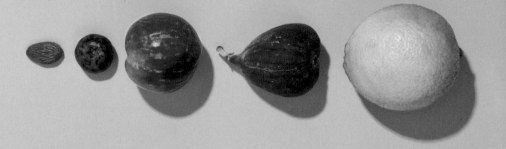

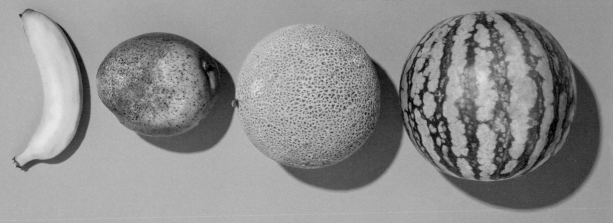

AUTHOR'S NOTE

Throughout this book, I refer to pregnant individuals as *women, mothers,* or other terms that indicate one particular gender. I realize that gender non-conforming people and those who identify as male can, do, and will continue to become pregnant. I use this language simply for ease of reading. The world is richer because of the great diversity among parents on this planet.

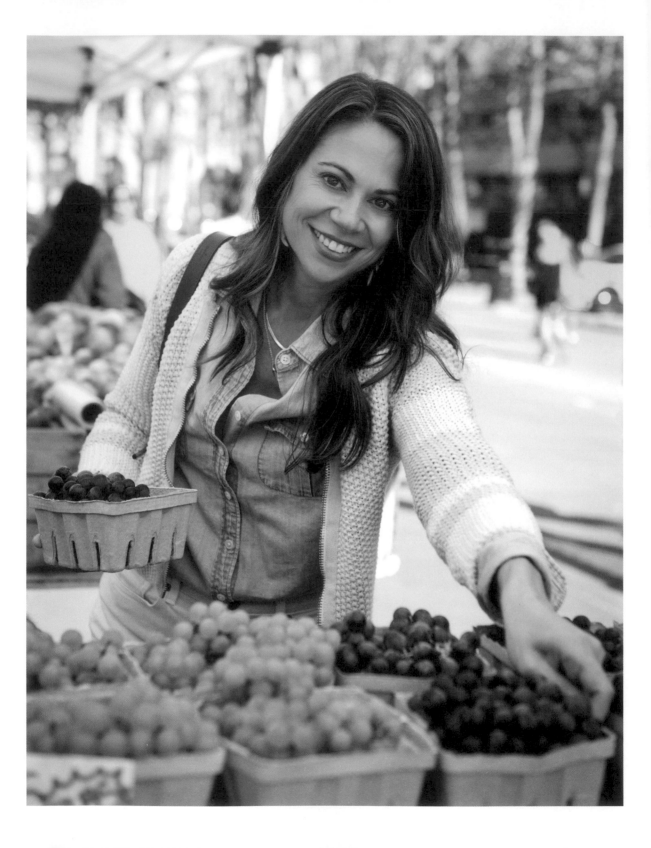

INTRODUCTION

Two months into my first pregnancy, the thought of food was too much to bear. While my pregnancy was medically fine, my appetite—like that of countless other women in their first trimester—was not. I knew I *had* to eat; it was vital to keep my body and my incredible growing baby nourished. I also knew that even though food might feel repulsive in the moment, it would—counterintuitively—make me feel better. So, I forced myself up, put on my robe and slippers, threw some cold water on my face, and headed into battle . . . uh, I mean, the kitchen. As I stared into the bright light of my open refrigerator, I had a bit of an epiphany. Here I was, a dictitian, an "expert," a speaker, an advisor, and a person with a bunch of letters after my name, yet I couldn't put my finger on one trusted source that would tell me how to eat during pregnancy.

Sure, as a registered dietitian-nutritionist, I knew what nutrients I needed and what foods would provide them, but I was missing how to make meals and snacks seem even remotely appealing and, more important, how they could make me *feel* better. I had recently had the "food conversation" with my OB, in which he outlined everything I shouldn't touch with a ten-foot pole, and before I even got off the table, my mind had inventoried everything to toss from my fridge. I walked out more nervous than reassured, second-guessing every food choice I had made or was about to make. I went home to a desk covered with different studies and articles about pregnancy health and nutrition—many clear and informative, but many contradictory and confusing. There *had* to be a better way.

I opened my laptop and tried to pull it all together. Now, this was 2014, so there were no momfluencers or overly polished day-in-the-life TikToks outlining how to master pregnancy and childbirth. There was just a *lot* of dense information coming at me from every corner of the globe, and over the next few months, I sorted through much of it. I read books, blogs, and articles. I spoke to many, many people, both experts and people who had been pregnant at some point. I asked my doctor questions—probably too many. I heard some helpful advice, but much of it was conflicting, out-of-date, or anecdotal ("My aunt's cousin's best friend drank wine every day of her pregnancy, and her kids are fine!"). Way too much of it shamed or scared me, adding a heavy dose of soon-to-be-mom guilt into the smoothie of pregnancy emotions. What I needed was one source—a go-to that would help me satisfy my cravings, ease my nausea, and put my food fears to rest. I couldn't find it.

I was frustrated and finally threw my hands up and decided to disregard the advice from all corners and go with what felt good. Things got better . . . sort of. I went from not wanting to drink water to craving my childhood comfort meal every day: roast chicken and potatoes. (My husband can't even look at roast chicken anymore.) I powered through some bumps in the road, from failing my first one-hour glucose tolerance test to becoming anemic, and I learned some valuable firsthand lessons. My kitchen turned back into just another room instead of a source of constant anxiety. But I knew all along that it could have been better, that my learning curve and relationship to food should have been *much* easier.

Then I gave birth to my son, Julian, and like so many other parents, I forgot about myself because life was now all about him. As I breastfed and pumped during my fourth trimester (and beyond), my entire focus was on eating to provide nourishment to this beautiful, healthy, insatiable boy. A few years later, I got pregnant with my daughter, Remi. I'd done all the research and had carried a child to term, yet I was back at square one. I knew every pregnancy is different, but I was surprised at *how* different it was. Still, I was dealing with the same issues around food—i.e., not knowing what to eat to support and satisfy my growing body and baby.

It was more apparent than ever that there wasn't one indispensable, easy-to-follow, nonscary resource for parents-to-be about food and nutrition. Eating is challenging enough during pregnancy because of morning sickness, exhaustion, and cravings, and adding in the "dangers" of foods to avoid makes everything so much worse. Do you really need to say no to soft cheese and sushi? Just how much coffee is too much? We already have enough on our shoulders (and bellies), so we don't need to make food an additional burden. Food should empower you. Food should be *fun*.

I've made it through two pregnancies, two books, thousands of happy clients, and a lot of hindsight. I've had moments that I handled reactively instead of proactively, saying "I wish I had known that!" or "Why didn't someone tell me?" I've seen pregnant people and parents struggling, overwhelmed with information and advice, terrified they were doing the wrong thing. I want to offer a resource that is helpful, informative, simple, and fun—something to make your pregnancy and beyond just a little easier.

At its core, this book's purpose is to remove a massive amount of stress and give you the tools to have a joyful pregnancy. It's intended to be a comprehensive resource (get out your highlighters and sticky notes!) for mamas-to-be (and their support teams) to ensure you are getting the right nutrition and foods to support your pregnancy, your health, and your mental well-being. There are over forty recipes and variations that will fortify you day by day, week by week, trimester by trimester. I'm not one to make everything from scratch or spend hours in the kitchen every day, so many of these are recipes anyone can make, and quickly. Some may take a tad longer but are still easy to follow. I've organized the book by trimester, as your body, your baby, your mindset, and your lifestyle require different things depending on which stage you're at. I'll cover everything from how to stock your pantry to what key vitamins and nutrients you need, when you need them, and how to get them. I'll address allergens, preparing your body for delivery, and healing postpartum. Just know that nothing is mandatory, because tastes and relationships with food vary greatly. Treat this book as a guide, not a map.

I want to remove the weight of food from your shoulders. My goal is to not only make your pregnancy as smooth as possible but also set you up for success long after you've delivered your bundle of joy. I want to equip you with the most up-to-date information told in the most loving way *and* give you some great recipes that will nourish you and your baby for the next ten months, and many more to come.

Thank you for putting your trust in me. I'm so excited to go on this journey with you.

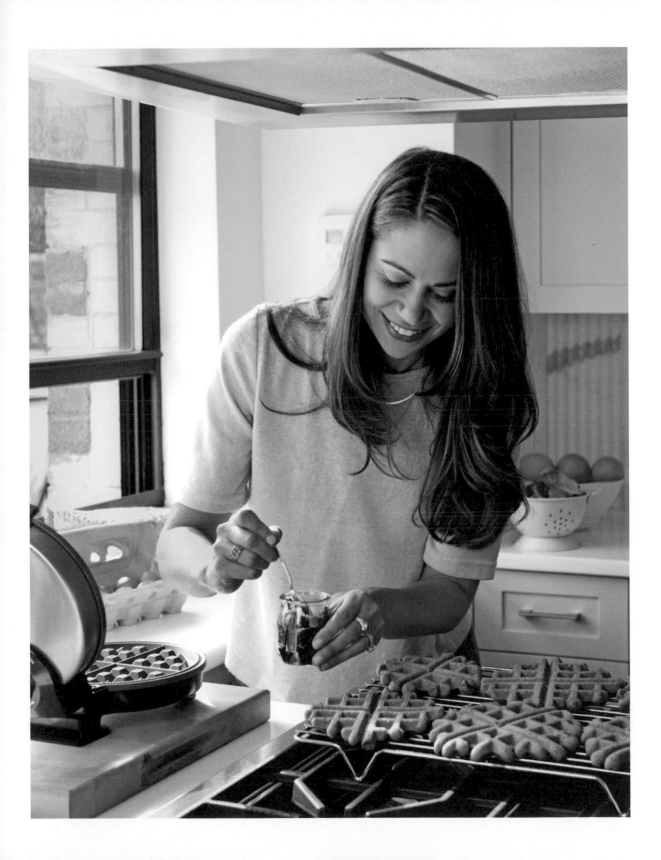

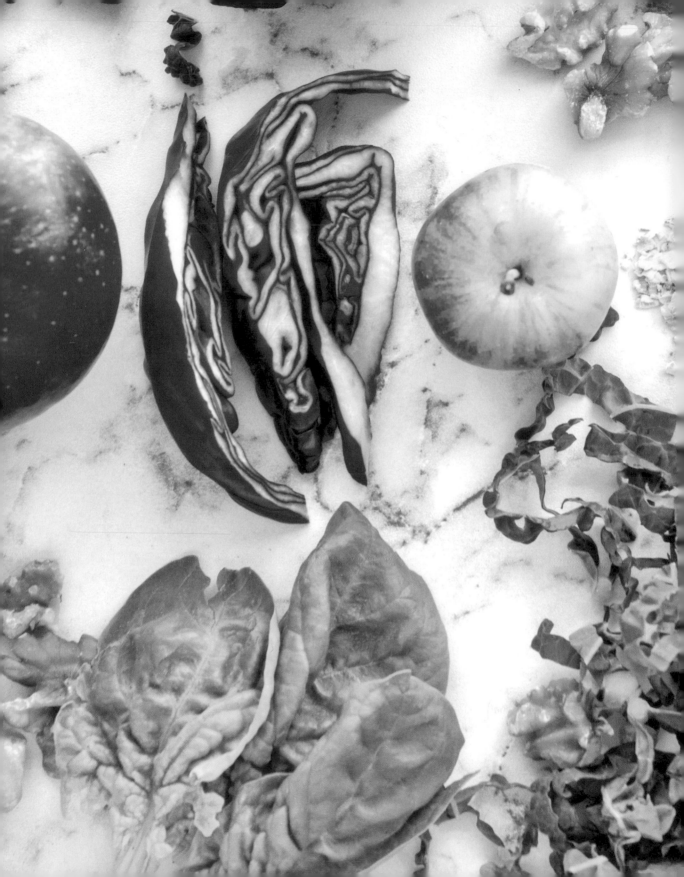

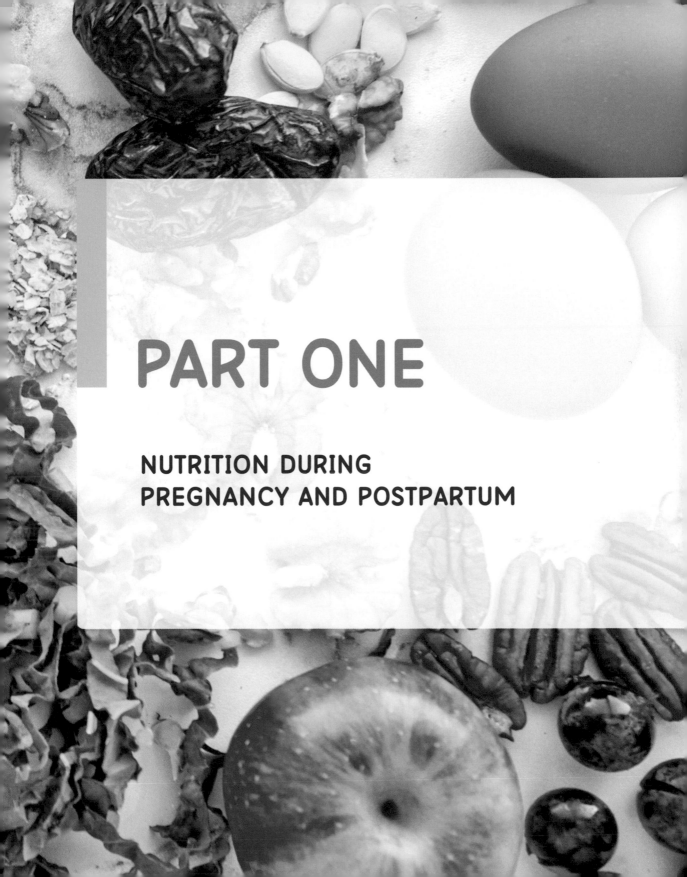

PART ONE

NUTRITION DURING PREGNANCY AND POSTPARTUM

SECTION ONE: THE FIRST TRIMESTER

First, congratulations are in order. You're pregnant! Amazing! Whatever journey you took to get here—long, short, complicated, or easy—this is an incredible moment, so pause, take a breath, and cherish it.

Now, let's get down to business. Just like millions of other women, you are probably experiencing a range of emotions, and your head may be spinning over things you need to do (or not do). If not, that's cool too. Regardless of how you're feeling, I know you're being bombarded with a ton of information from every direction. Much of it is about food. There's what you should and shouldn't eat and what you can eat a little of . . . but not too much. You may receive doom and gloom from even your biggest cheerleaders, and you'll *definitely* hear the personal views of every person in your life. My local baker told me to eat dates so I'd go into labor, then handed me a bag of them. Fear not. I am going to simplify and walk you through everything related to pregnancy nutrition, and if I do my job right, I'm going to make food enjoyable for you for the full four trimesters (yes, *four*) and beyond.

So, let's start at the beginning: your first trimester. Over the next eighty-eight pages, I am going to cover what's going on in your body and with your little one, how early pregnancy affects your appetite, and the nutrition you'll need for these first twelve weeks. I'll also cover prenatal supplements, nutrients you and your growing baby need, and, of course, the foods that you should be careful of or cut out, with a basis in scientific evidence, not random emails from your aunt. This first section sets the stage for you to understand the whys and hows of what to expect in later pregnancy.

Then, we'll get right to it and go grocery shopping. I know you're on the waiting list for the eco-friendly expandable crib du jour that your child will use until they're a teenager, and I promise I'll make shopping for food feel like a less intimidating part of pregnancy too. In fact, I've done half the work with a simple yet comprehensive pantry list on page 80.

Let's get started, because that baby is waiting for no one.

CHAPTER 1

YOUR CHANGING BODY AND DEVELOPING BABY

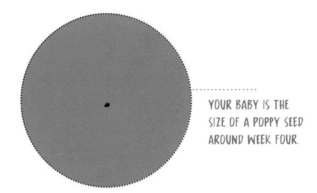

YOUR BABY IS THE SIZE OF A POPPY SEED AROUND WEEK FOUR.

I'm not going to sugarcoat things: the first trimester can be rough. Barring any unforeseen complications later on, it will most likely be the most difficult point of your pregnancy. (I want to emphasize "might." Many women have problem-free first trimesters, with only a gorgeous glow as a side effect.)

From the moment of conception, your body goes through major changes, both physically and physiologically, and you may begin to feel them pretty quickly. When I was newly pregnant with my son, I lost my appetite and was exhausted all the time. Then, with my daughter, I was starving and exhausted, and my face broke out. Oh, the joys! Other women feel like an alien has invaded their body, and they experience morning sickness, aches and pains, and other fun stuff that we don't need to go into right now. (If you know, you know.) I hope you're one of the lucky ones. Everyone's body is different and there is no *right* way to feel.

The first trimester is the time to really listen to your body—and above all to respect it. One minute you may be starving with an urgency you've never felt before, the next repulsed by the thought of food. You may experience acid reflux, and you may get so full so quickly that you cannot take another bite. You may feel like a bottomless pit. Whatever your experience, treat yourself *kindly*. Your body has a whole new set of needs, and it's depending on you to nourish and care for it, for your sake and your baby's. No pressure, right?

Unfortunately, this is also the time when parents-to-be are bombarded by all the don'ts. Don't eat sushi, don't drink alcohol, and *definitely* don't even think about having that second cup of coffee. I'll cover all that information—and misinformation—in a second. The key through line here is that all the changes in your body and during your baby's development significantly impact what you want to eat, what you need to eat, and in some cases even how you eat it. I personally found that being fed frozen grapes by my husband while lying in bed watching a bad rom-com was the best way for me to deal with morning sickness.

Before we jump into the subjects of pregnancy nutrition and delicious, nourishing food, I want to put on my lab coat and give a brief overview of what's happening in your body right now, as well as some major developments that your baby undergoes during the first trimester. It's important to understand the why behind the cravings, needs, and recommendations you'll be reading about in the rest of this chapter.

HORMONES IN THE FIRST TRIMESTER

One day everything is normal, and the next day . . . A WHOLE NEW WORLD. The nausea, fatigue, cravings (or lack of cravings), brain fog, or whatever you endure during the first trimester is due to those fun chemicals inside your body: hormones. In particular, three hormones that ramp up and put your changing body on high alert during the first trimester:

- **Estrogen:** Estrogen is responsible for a lot of the growth during pregnancy. It builds up your uterine lining, boosts the growth of the uterus, and stimulates the development of your baby's organs. Estrogen skyrockets in the first trimester, and it is likely responsible for a lot of the nausea you may feel.

- **Progesterone:** At the start of the second month of pregnancy, progesterone—which also helps the uterus expand—takes the lead. Progesterone essentially signals your body's systems to slow down and relax, which accentuates some of the more uncomfortable feelings, like fatigue and nausea . . . and more fatigue. Coupled with the increase in estrogen, it can also make you feel a little (or a lot) moody and emotional.

- **Human chorionic gonadotropin (hCG):** When you see that second blue line or happy face pop up on your home pregnancy test, you've witnessed the work of hCG. It's the hormone that pregnancy tests monitor, and it rises until it peaks between weeks nine and twelve. HCG amps up the production of estrogen and progesterone, and it can cause all kinds of early pregnancy symptoms, including moodiness, light spotting, breast soreness, bloating, and—you guessed it—nausea.

YOUR BABY'S DEVELOPMENT

It's hard to put into words what you'll see on that first sonogram. Your baby is developing, well, *everything* they need to grow and thrive. While I'll cover their nutritional needs later, here's a brief overview of the developmental milestones in the first three months.

- **Heart:** Your baby's heart begins to beat around week five or six, which is generally the highlight of the first sonogram. At the end of the first trimester, it is the size of a pea.

- **Neural tube:** Around week six, your baby's neural tube has formed. The neural tube will lead to the development of the brain and spinal cord.

- **Brain:** By week seven, the brain is forming.

- **Toes, nose, ears, and arms:** By weeks nine and ten, your baby has a small—but recognizable—set of appendages. Baby has fingers, ears (though they can't hear), and a teeny tiny nose.

- **Intestines:** By week twelve, your baby has intestines in their abdomen.

That's a lot of growing for someone so small, and all those changes your baby is going through affect your body, and vice versa—the nutrition you take in can help them develop. Equally important, good nutrition in the first trimester can help *you* feel good (or, at least, not terrible). The next chapter will show you why and how.

CHAPTER 2

TESTS, SUPPLEMENTS, AND YOUR FIRST TRIMESTER NUTRITIONAL NEEDS

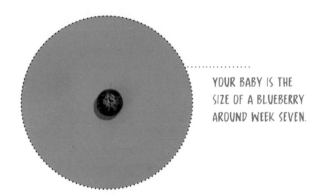

YOUR BABY IS THE SIZE OF A BLUEBERRY AROUND WEEK SEVEN.

Now that we've covered why you feel the way you do and what's happening with you and baby, let's get into what you should do to set yourself up for a healthy pregnancy and ensure you get all the nutrition you need in the way that works best for you. A few of these tips are above and beyond what the doctor might order, but never fear—the point is to put you at ease and to set you up on a sustainable, actionable path for a healthy pregnancy.

KEY NUTRIENTS DURING PREGNANCY

First things first. What are the must-have nutrients for every expectant mother and her baby? What's good for mom is good for baby, and what is good for baby is good for mom, but it's helpful to know why to focus on certain nutrients. Your nutritional needs change from the moment of conception, and understanding what your body needs even after pregnancy, when you're nursing or simply recovering, is key.

Use this chart to get oriented about food, eating, and how to build up your nutrient stores. Note that it refers to key vitamins and minerals, as well as some of the most common food-based essentials, like choline, that you should concentrate on throughout all three trimesters. I'll dive deeper into many of these nutrients, as well as other recommendations (like probiotics), later on. In addition, know that often food isn't enough to provide all the vitamins and minerals your body requires during pregnancy; that's where prenatal vitamins enter the picture. I'll discuss supplements later in this chapter (see page 26).

NUTRIENT	HOW IT HELPS MOM	HOW IT HELPS BABY	FOOD SOURCES
Folate (B_9)	Promotes heart health Supports the immune system Balances mood Builds healthy blood cells	Supports normal neural tube development Forms red blood cells Promotes cell growth and function	Asparagus, spinach, broccoli, lentils, Brussels sprouts, kale, eggs, artichokes, avocados, and beets
Vitamin B_6	Reduces nausea Balances blood sugar Stabilizes mood Helps the body utilize protein	Aids in your baby's brain and nervous system development	Poultry, fish, bananas, avocados, sunflower seeds, chickpeas, leafy greens, and organ meat

NUTRIENT	HOW IT HELPS MOM	HOW IT HELPS BABY	FOOD SOURCES
Vitamin B_{12}	Supports cognitive health, healthy metabolism, and good energy levels	Helps develop the nervous system, brain, DNA synthesis, and red blood cells Works with folate to support neural tube development	Poultry, red meat, organ meat, salmon, sardines, shellfish, full-fat dairy like Greek yogurt, cottage cheese, and hard cheeses
Vitamin C	Supports the immune system Prevents cell damage Maintains a healthy metabolism Builds connective tissue	Helps developing tendons, bones, skin, and cartilage Promotes a healthy birth weight Supports immune function	Oranges, nectarines, lemons, kiwi, red and yellow bell peppers, broccoli, strawberries, kale, and tomatoes
Choline	Assists with brain processing Good for cardiovascular health	Supports brain and cognition development Helps to prevent neural tube deficiency	Eggs (the best source, as two eggs contain over half your daily needs), liver, pork, beef, salmon, cod, cruciferous vegetables, and beans
Docosa-hexaenoic Acid (DHA)	Promotes cardiovascular health Reduces inflammation Improves mood Improves eye functioning	Essential for brain and vision development Supports a healthy immune system	Seafood (like salmon, tuna, sardines, herring, anchovies, and cooked shellfish), grass-fed meats, pasture-raised eggs, and algae (the only vegan source)

NUTRIENT	HOW IT HELPS MOM	HOW IT HELPS BABY	FOOD SOURCES
Vitamin A	Supports immune function and skin health Maintains thyroid function Builds the placenta Repairs uterine tissue postpartum Supports milk supply	Assists development of eyes and ears Supports full-term gestation and optimal birth weight Helps develop strong teeth and bones	There are two types: · Preformed vitamin A (or retinol): found in animal products like eggs, full-fat dairy, and liver · Provitamin A (or carotene): plant-based, found in orange and yellow fruits and veggies like carrots and sweet potatoes Consume both forms, but know that the plant-based ones (carotene) are less ideal sources as they need to first get converted to the active form, retinol.
Vitamin D$_3$	Strengthens bones Builds immunity Reduces inflammation Maintains a healthy blood pressure Reduces risk of gestational diabetes and preeclampsia	Supports bone and teeth growth May help prevent childhood asthma, ADHD, and some autoimmune disorders Supports a healthy immune system and respiratory function	The best source of D$_3$ is sunlight. It's very hard to get enough from food, but include salmon, sardines, mackerel, and egg yolks.

NUTRIENT	HOW IT HELPS MOM	HOW IT HELPS BABY	FOOD SOURCES
Vitamin E	Protects the body against damage from free radicals Maintains healthy skin and normal cardiac function May help prevent miscarriage, preeclampsia, and hypertension	Protects the body against damage from free radicals Enhances fetal growth and function	Sunflower seeds, almonds, peanuts, broccoli, avocados, salmon, kiwi, and mangoes
Vitamin K	Serves as a helper nutrient for vitamin D and calcium Promotes bone health Balances blood sugar Helps with blood clotting Protects skin elasticity	Strengthens bones and teeth Promotes healthy blood clotting Supports cardiovascular health	Leafy greens, full-fat dairy, and eggs
Calcium	Maintains strong bones Decreases the risk of preeclampsia and high blood pressure in pregnancy	Builds strong teeth and bones Develops a healthy heart, strong muscles, and a functioning nervous system	Dairy sources: full-fat yogurt, cottage cheese, cheese Nondairy sources: kale, bok choy, fish with bones found in canned sardines and canned wild salmon, sesame seeds and tahini, almonds, and tofu

NUTRIENT	HOW IT HELPS MOM	HOW IT HELPS BABY	FOOD SOURCES
Iodine	Maintains healthy thyroid function	Develops the brain, nervous system, and thyroid Supports healthy birth weight	Full-fat dairy, seaweed (like kelp noodles or flakes and nori snacks), shellfish, cod, and eggs
Iron	Supports placental growth Deficiency increases the risk of preterm birth, low birth weight, preeclampsia, and impaired thyroid function	Plays an important role in fetal development Forms healthy red blood cells Develops the nervous system Deficiency is associated with lower cognition and fetal growth	Heme iron (animal protein and well absorbed): red meat, poultry, fish (like cooked oysters and canned sardines), liver, and other organ meat Nonheme iron (plant-based and not well absorbed): green leafy vegetables like cooked spinach and kale, beans, lentils, tofu, and pumpkin seeds
Magnesium	Works with vitamin D, vitamin K, and calcium to optimize bone health Prevents leg cramps and high blood pressure Keeps you regular Deficiency has also been linked to gestational diabetes, preeclampisa, and preterm birth	Prevents small birth weight Supports proper fetal development, including strong bones and teeth Supports a healthy nervous system	Pumpkin seeds, sesame seeds, sunflower seeds, cashews, almonds, seaweed, spinach, bone broth, and dark chocolate

NUTRIENT	HOW IT HELPS MOM	HOW IT HELPS BABY	FOOD SOURCES
Selenium	Protects the body from free radical damage Assists with immune function Offsets the effects of mercury consumption	Assists with cognitive development Lowers the risk of preterm birth	Brazil nuts, tuna (canned light or skipjack), salmon, sardines, eggs, cottage cheese, sunflower seeds, grass-fed meats, poultry, and grains
Zinc	Helps regulate mood during pregnancy and postpartum Aids in optimum thyroid function Optimizes immune system	Assists in DNA and protein synthesis Supports a healthy immune system	Oysters are the best source (consume cooked if pregnant); otherwise, red meat, organ meats, pork and chicken (dark meat), and eggs are great sources. Vegetarian sources include legumes like baked beans and chickpeas, nuts, seeds, and whole grains. Vegetarian sources of zinc are not absorbed as well.

THE IMPORTANCE OF BLOOD WORK

One of the things I wish I'd done before both of my pregnancies was to get thorough blood work done. My doctor didn't recommend it, and I assumed that because I was healthy and had never had any issues with nutrient levels, I didn't need it.

Today, I know that even if you *feel* fine, you might not *be* fine. A significant number of women go into pregnancy deficient in at least one essential nutrient, so it's crucial to have a good sense of your body's baseline. Are you a vegetarian (which might affect your iron levels)? Have you been on hormonal birth control for years? (More on this later.) Do you have digestive issues? Have you occasionally had high blood sugar? Gather this information so you know where your greatest needs are.

Early blood work can also help you avoid common side effects. Even if your prenatal levels were perfect, they can dip when you're expecting (I became anemic and vitamin D deficient). Low levels of essential nutrients may lead to side effects as minor as exhaustion or as major as anemia or gestational diabetes. With that baby inside you, your body simply needs certain nutrients more than others—and more than it did before—and not getting (or getting too much of) them can lead to complications or discomfort.

You may be asking, "Wait, if blood work is so important, why isn't it standard for prenatal care?" I'll be honest, I wonder that all the time, and while at the moment I'm not going down the rabbit hole of our health-care system, I will say this: You are the best advocate for yourself and your baby. Period. Full stop. If your provider doesn't bring it up, ask to have your levels tested. The results will give you that first bit of insight into what you're feeling and how things will play out during pregnancy and postpartum. Maybe your levels are great. Phew! Then you can focus your attention on other things. Or maybe the report comes back with a few issues. Then you can nip them in the bud by tweaking your habits or diet and keep an eye out for problems down the road.

I recommend monitoring key nutrient levels in your blood to determine if you're meeting the necessary requirements during pregnancy. I do want to acknowledge that some are outside the blood panels a doctor typically prescribes and may or may not be covered, so make sure to call your insurance provider ahead of time to make sure they don't require preauthorization or reject the claims altogether. Do the best you can. Don't stress about anything that's out of your control. If you can swing it, great. If not, no biggie. Knowing which vitamins and nutrients are the most important is half the battle.

Here are the nutrient levels to test for:

- **Iron (ferritin, hematocrit, hemoglobin):** Iron needs are one and a half times higher in pregnancy, when a woman produces more red blood cells to support the growth of the baby and the placenta. That means you go from needing eighteen milligrams a day to twenty-seven milligrams a day. Roughly 40 percent of pregnant women worldwide are deficient in iron, especially during the third trimester (I was in both my pregnancies). Severe deficiency can lead to anemia, a lack of red blood cells in the body that may increase the risks of your baby having low birth weight and delayed neurocognitive development. Your OB will likely screen for anemia during your first prenatal labs and then again midpregnancy. But if at any point you feel particularly weak, can't maintain body warmth, have shortness of breath, become pale, or have a rapid heartbeat or heart palpitations, let your doctor know because it's worth getting your iron checked out.

- **Vitamin B$_{12}$:** B$_{12}$ requirements are also much higher in pregnancy. Adequate B$_{12}$ influences fetal brain and nervous system development, and low levels have been linked to preterm birth, early miscarriage, preeclampsia, and in the baby, neural tube defects and a small size for gestational age. Really low levels may also increase the baby's risk of heart problems later in childhood. A deficiency in pregnancy is common, though, and it's easy to both prevent and fix. Women who follow a vegan or vegetarian diet, who have been on birth control for years, and/or who have used a lot of antacids due to heartburn or other gastrointestinal (GI) issues (like celiac disease) are at a much higher risk of being B$_{12}$ deficient. In fact, research shows that 62 percent of vegetarian pregnant women are deficient in B$_{12}$, and 38 percent of all pregnant women are B$_{12}$ deficient at delivery. Read: B$_{12}$ is something to monitor throughout pregnancy, not just at the beginning.

BIRTH CONTROL AND VITAMIN DEFICIENCY

When I learned that being on hormonal birth control could deplete the body's store of key nutrients—especially for those trying to conceive or who are pregnant—it was a huge aha moment. Most of us are never warned of this at *any* point when we are on the pill.

Birth control pills can deplete the body of key nutrients like B_{12}, B_6, riboflavin, magnesium, folate, selenium, vitamins C, D, and E, and zinc. In fact, a recent study showed that women who go off the pill have levels of vitamin D that are up to 20 percent lower than women who have never been on it! Low levels in mom can also lead to low levels in baby.

Like so much in life, taking the pill is a trade-off, and the benefits may outweigh the side effects for you. Being deficient in certain nutrients may not lead to health issues. If you were on the pill for years before getting pregnant, get your blood work done so you can see where you are and then focus on building those nutrient stores back up.

· **Vitamin D:** Deficiency is common in general and even more so in pregnancy, which may put you or your baby at greater risk for preeclampsia, gestational diabetes, or low birth weight. We typically get vitamin D from the sun, so it's not something you can easily add more of through diet alone. Ask your OB to test your levels at the start of pregnancy and a few times throughout. Most labs will say that you are within range with a number of at least thirty nanograms per milliliter. However, "in range" is not the same as optimal, and I recommend your levels be closer to forty nanograms per milliliter. Depending on what your labs say and how much vitamin D is in your prenatal vitamin, you may need to supplement with between 2,000 and 5,000 IUs/day, or more. Vitamin D is fat soluble, meaning you can have too much, so test your levels after taking it for a month or two to make sure you're still in that optimal range.

· **Hemoglobin A1c/Fasting Blood Glucose:** An A1c test offers some information as to what has been going on with your blood sugar in the past three months. Since you don't get screened for gestational diabetes until weeks twenty-four to twenty-eight in your pregnancy (or earlier if you're considered of "advanced maternal age," which is typically thirty-five and up), having a baseline awareness of your blood sugar levels will help you understand whether or not to focus on regulation. Research has shown that high hemoglobin A1c (anything above 5.7) in the first trimester predicts gestational diabetes. If you get early test results that indicate that you're at risk, don't worry. You now have the opportunity to be proactive about your health from the start. I discuss *a lot* more about foods that can balance your blood sugar in chapter 6.

PREEXISTING DIABETES AND PREGNANCY

It's estimated that 1 to 2 percent of women who become pregnant each year have type 1 or type 2 diabetes. That doesn't sound like a huge percentage, but given that there are over 3.6 million live births in the US a year, that's up to seventy-two thousand women. I hope that all of these women have a doctor (especially an endocrinologist) they trust, but a registered dietitian can also be a huge help in managing the particular nutritional concerns of pregnancy and diabetes. Many insurance plans cover a few visits with a dietitian, so, if you have diabetes or prediabetes, it's worth doing the research.

· **Thyroid Panel:** You want to make sure your thyroid is functioning normally for many reasons, in particular for your baby's brain development, which the mother's thyroid hormones control via the placenta. Adequate thyroid levels are crucial during pregnancy, yet only thyroid-stimulating hormone (TSH) and thyroxine (Free T4) are routinely screened for. If you have high thyroid antibodies (TPOAb or TgAb), you are at risk of thyroid issues postpartum, so I encourage you to advocate for a full thyroid panel that includes the following:

   · TSH (this is the most common test in pregnancy)
   · Free T4 (this is also pretty standard)
   · Free T3: triiodothyronine
   · Reverse T3: reverse triiodothyronine

- TPOAb: thyroid peroxidase antibodies
- TgAb: thyroglobulin antibodies

As I said, there are heaps of other blood tests available, but these are the key ones during the first trimester. And for those of you squeamish about needles, they are all quick, easy, and only require a small amount of blood. You'll be in and out of the lab in no time.

PRENATAL SUPPLEMENTS

I remember sitting in my doctor's office during my first pregnancy and bringing up prenatal vitamins. As someone who loves the science of nutrients, I geeked out. What should I be taking, how much should I be taking, and *why*? Instead of a rousing discussion, though, all I got was a simple "Yes, take a prenatal."

"Should I take an extra vitamin D supplement?" I asked.

The answer was "Sure, why not? Do you need it? *I* don't think so, but it can't hurt."

It didn't exactly leave me feeling confident.

When it comes to supplements, most of us don't know what to look for. Most of us just walk into the drugstore and grab the first prenatal we see or (best-case scenario) pick one based on the recommendation of a friend. You've probably already spent hours researching the best bottles, pacifiers, strollers, and STEM toys, but it's time to get back to basics.

Let's start first with the why of prenatals. The physical transformation that you're going through alters your physiology as your body turns itself into a caretaker for the incredible growing being inside of you. You're going to require different types and different quantities of the nutrients you're used to. These will all go to support your baby's development and your well-being. While some schools of thought say you don't need to supplement in pregnancy if you are following a healthy diet, the fact of the matter is that your needs are a lot higher now, and the extra help and support a few capsules can provide far outweigh trying to force food down that might not appeal. Food is also a big part of the equation, but prenatals will ensure you're getting what you need.

Just below, you'll find a quick Q and A about prenatals, based on the questions I had when I was pregnant and that my clients frequently ask. I've also created a chart that goes over what to look for in a prenatal and why so you don't get overwhelmed standing in the vitamin aisle. Then we'll delve deeper into the nutrients that deserve extra attention and the special needs of those with specific diets (vegans and vegetarians in particular).

PRENATAL Q&A
Do I really need a prenatal vitamin?

YES. In an ideal world you could meet all your nutritional needs through food alone, but even those who eat a perfect nutrient-dense diet are probably not getting everything they need while pregnant. A prenatal is a really good way to ensure a baseline of nutrient absorption. It's in no way a cure-all, but it forms a strong nutritional foundation. Recent studies show that your body's requirements for many essential nutrients are *much* higher than previously thought and that a lot of pregnant women are deficient. Taking into account your personal medical history, what medicines you may have been on, etc., may mean that you need extra support.

Is a prenatal the only vitamin I need?

Unfortunately, no, as not all prenatal vitamins are created equal. Many only include the bare minimum amounts of nutrients, which are based on the percent of daily values recommended by the Food and Drug Administration (FDA). These levels prevent severe deficiency but don't necessarily focus on optimal nutrition. Some brands include lower-quality forms of certain nutrients, often because they are cheaper, that aren't as bioavailable (meaning your body metabolizes a high percent, making their nutrients quickly available to your cells). Some don't include certain necessary nutrients at all! Check out the chart beginning on page 30 for the key nutrients to look for and in what form. Then we'll dive into other supplements that may be worth taking.

What's the best way to take prenatal supplements?

Ideally, it's best to take your supplements with food, as it helps with absorption and reduces side effects like nausea. Aim for late morning or around lunch because many people experience nausea taking them early in the morning, when the stomach acid isn't performing at its peak. If your prenatal requires multiple pills a day, spread them out (some with every meal or split over two meals) as you can only absorb so many nutrients at once. Avoid taking your prenatal with dinner or near bedtime, since some of the vitamins (like methylated B vitamins) are energizing and can interfere with sleep. They may also lead to acid reflux. But, like anything, experiment and find what works best for you. Everyone responds differently.

How many prenatals should I take a day?

Once upon a time, prenatals came as one megasized pill a day, but there are now a lot of different brands in the market that require multiple pills per day—some as many as eight pills a day. While the prenatals with more pills do often provide more nutrients, they might not be right for you. The key is to find a brand that works for your needs and that you can consistently take.

Can you switch prenatals?

Absolutely! Find the one that works best for you, but don't mix and match. Give each brand a few days or a week, and if it's not working for you (meaning you have unpleasant side effects, feel like you're spending too much money, or see no change in your blood levels if there was a deficiency), make the switch.

Are there any side effects?

For some, yes, and for others, not at all. Common side effects include constipation (from iron), nausea (from pill size or additives), and bloating or gas (perhaps from the omega-3 fatty acid DHA). If any of these are making you feel worse instead of better, try a new prenatal.

I can't stand the thought of swallowing even one of those pills. What should I do?

I totally get that, and the good news is you have options. First up: chewable prenatals. While they are not my first choice, as they typically don't contain the highest amounts of vitamins and minerals, and often contain sugar and additives to make them chewy and sweet, they could be a good plan B. Remember, in pregnancy as in life, the perfect should never be the enemy of the good.

Second, there are high-quality powder and liquid prenatals on the market. The downside to powders is that you have to add them to yogurt, a smoothie, or some other food, and that can alter the taste. Liquid vitamins are highly bioavailable and help a lot of women avoid the nausea that comes from taking vitamins first thing in the morning. This can be huge, especially when you already have morning sickness. The main downside is that they can be pricey. But if they're feeling good for your body, they may be worth the extra cost.

How do I know if what I am taking is high quality?

Here's a dirty little secret. I can go to a beach, fill a bottle with sand, and call it vitamins—and no one can stop me. The FDA does not test or certify vitamins like it does food and medications, and the industry is *largely* unregulated. That's why it's more important than ever to buy from brands that—ideally—have partnered with third-party research organizations, tested their products in clinical trials, and don't contain fillers and unnecessary additives (like sugar!). A strong brand tells customers the truth about its manufacturing processes and supports the claims it makes on the label with hard science and testing done by third-party organizations (the resources section on page 274 can guide you).

I also consider a high-quality prenatal to be one that contains the optimal amount of the key nutrients in the most ideal form for you. Before you go shopping, refer to the prenatal chart that follows, make sure the one you pick contains those nutrients, and take a formulation that boosts your health and doesn't lead to too many side effects.

NUTRIENT	WHAT FORM TO LOOK FOR	RECOMMENDED DIETARY ALLOWANCE (RDA) OR ADEQUATE INTAKE (AI)	DO MOST PRENATALS CONTAIN ENOUGH?
Folate (B_9)	Look for activated forms like L-methylfolate, 5-methyltetrahydro-folate, L-5-MTHF, or 5-MTHF. You want to avoid folic acid, as it is a synthetic version of folate and is not well utilized by the body in many women.	Pregnancy: 600 mcg Lactation: 500 mcg	Most likely, yes.
Vitamin B_6	Look for the activated form, pyridoxal 5-phosphate.	Pregnancy: 1.9 mg Lactation: 2 mg	You may need an additional supplement of 25 to 50 mg twice a day if you have severe nausea. Start on the lower end especially if your prenatal already contains B_6. Many pregnant women go into pregnancy low in B_6 as hormonal birth control depletes your stores.

NUTRIENT	WHAT FORM TO LOOK FOR	RECOMMENDED DIETARY ALLOWANCE (RDA) OR ADEQUATE INTAKE (AI)	DO MOST PRENATALS CONTAIN ENOUGH?
Vitamin B_{12}	Look for the types called adenosylcobalamin or methylcobalamin. These are methylated—or activated—B_{12} that your body can more easily metabolize.	Pregnancy: 2.6 mcg Lactation: 2.8 mcg	They should, but you may need more if you are a vegan/vegetarian, have been on the pill for many years, have taken lots of antacids in the past, or have lower levels based on your blood work. For some women, oral B_{12} supplements don't always help to bring levels up as effectively as injections and food sources of B_{12}.
Vitamin C		Pregnancy: Under 19 years: 80 mg 19+ years: 85 mg Lactation: Under 19 years: 115 mg 19+ years: 120 mg	Most likely, yes.

NUTRIENT	WHAT FORM TO LOOK FOR	RECOMMENDED DIETARY ALLOWANCE (RDA) OR ADEQUATE INTAKE (AI)	DO MOST PRENATALS CONTAIN ENOUGH?
Vitamin A	Ideally, look for a combination of both the active form—retinol, typically listed as retinyl palmitate—and beta-carotene. This is especially important if you don't consume meat.	Pregnancy: Under 19 years: 750 mcg 19+ years: 770 mcg Lactation: Under 19 years: 1,200 mcg RAE 19+ years: 1,300 mcg RAE	High-dose supplementation of preformed vitamin A or retinol has been linked to toxicity. You may see supplements leave out this form and use only beta-carotene, which for vegetarians is not ideal. You do not need to worry about toxicity with food sources of vitamin A.
Vitamin D_3	Be sure to look for it in D_3 form (versus D_2), as it more closely mimics the D you get from the sun, and your body absorbs it better.	600 IUs (international units)	Probably not. Even though the RDA is 600 IUs/day, most women need closer to 2,000 to 4,000 IU. Most prenatals contain only 400 to 800 IUs. Additional supplementing will probably be necessary, depending on your blood work and how much D_3 your body absorbs.

NUTRIENT	WHAT FORM TO LOOK FOR	RECOMMENDED DIETARY ALLOWANCE (RDA) OR ADEQUATE INTAKE (AI)	DO MOST PRENATALS CONTAIN ENOUGH?
Vitamin E		Pregnancy: 15 mg Lactation: 19 mg	Most likely, yes.
Vitamin K	Look for vitamin K_1 and vitamin K_2. Ideally look for vitamin K_2 as menaquinone (MK-7). It is more bioavailable than other forms of K_2.	Pregnancy and lactation: Under 19 years: 75 mcg 19+ years: 90 mcg	Many prenatals contain K_1 rather than K_2. Aim to include plenty of full-fat dairy, eggs, and fermented foods like natto, miso, and sauerkraut if your prenatal does not have K_2.
Calcium		1,000 mg Recommendations don't increase in pregnancy, but your body absorbs almost double the amount of calcium in pregnancy.	Deficiency is not common. However, if you do not consume dairy, try to focus on other sources to get the extra you need from food. If you do need to supplement with extra calcium, make sure you take it separately from any iron as they compete for absorption.

NUTRIENT	WHAT FORM TO LOOK FOR	RECOMMENDED DIETARY ALLOWANCE (RDA) OR ADEQUATE INTAKE (AI)	DO MOST PRENATALS CONTAIN ENOUGH?
Iodine		The RDA for pregnant women is almost 50 percent higher than that for nonpregnant women. 220 mcg versus 150 mcg for nonpregnant women	The American Thyroid Association published a study that revealed that 58 percent of prenatals contain iodine, which means that 42 percent don't!
Iron	Look for iron bisglycinate (it is better absorbed with fewer side effects).	Iron needs increase from 18 mg to 27 mg in pregnancy, and the Centers for Disease Control (CDC) recommends you take 30 mg of iron a day while pregnant. Iron needs are highest in the third trimester, when blood volume peaks.	Not all prenatals contain iron, as needs are individualized and some women experience side effects from iron in supplement form. You will most likely need to supplement with iron if you are a vegetarian/vegan or have a history of anemia or heavy periods. Iron needs during pregnancy are one and a half times higher than when you're not pregnant, so be sure to review your blood levels.

NUTRIENT	WHAT FORM TO LOOK FOR	RECOMMENDED DIETARY ALLOWANCE (RDA) OR ADEQUATE INTAKE (AI)	DO MOST PRENATALS CONTAIN ENOUGH?
Magnesium	Look for magnesium glycinate or magnesium bisglycinate, which are the better-absorbed forms. Avoid magnesium oxalate and carbonate, and try magnesium citrate if you are constipated.	Aim for an intake of 300 to 500 mg.	They may not. Deficiency is very common in pregnancy.
Selenium		60 mcg	Many do not.
Zinc		Pregnancy: Under 19 years: 13 mg 19+ years: 11 mg Lactation: Under 19 years: 13 mg 19+ years: 12 mg	Most likely, yes.

Your prenatal should also include niacin, thiamin, riboflavin, pantothenic acid, copper, manganese, chromium, sodium, biotin, and potassium, so check the label on yours to make sure it contains them.

SUPPLEMENTING YOUR SUPPLEMENTS

As you can see, a good prenatal gives you a lot of bang for your buck, but it's not going to give you everything, especially at the levels you'll need. So, while I always recommend trying to limit what you're taking in supplement form (as opposed to getting from real food), there are a few additions to the supplement menu that you should consider. Yes, this may mean more pills, but you and your baby are worth it.

Omega-3 Fatty Acids

Omega-3 fatty acids are polyunsaturated fatty acids that are essential for your baby's brain and neurological development. They also support your baby's immune system, eye development, and cardiovascular health and protect you against postpartum depression. Outside of supplements, you can get a sufficient quantity of omega-3s from sources like salmon, tuna, sardines, herring, anchovies, shellfish, and algae. If you don't eat or aren't craving fish or seafood, you'll need to get it elsewhere. I recommend a combined DHA/EPA supplement, which is typically derived from fish oil. If you are vegetarian or vegan, know that most algae-based supplements contain DHA but not EPA, so please check the label carefully.

What are DHA and EPA? In addition to ALA, they make up the three types of omega-3s:

- **Docosahexaenoic acid (DHA) and Eicosapentaenoic Acid (EPA):** Both are derived from fish like salmon, tuna, herring, sardines, anchovies, and shellfish.

- **Alpha-linolenic acid (ALA):** ALA is found in plants (like flaxseed, chia seeds, walnuts, and more), and although it's healthy, it is not the most important form of omega for pregnant women.

While the recommended daily allowance for DHA is three hundred milligrams, a rule of thumb is that if you don't eat fish, can't bear to be around it during pregnancy, or don't get it at least twice a week, you should supplement, and that supplement should ideally contain both DHA and EPA. Refrigerate the bottle to keep it fresh. You may also want to check to see whether a product is approved by the International Fish Oil Standards program (a third-party testing and quality-control organization) or look for the GOED (Global Organization for EPA and DHA omega-3s) quality seal on the label.

Finally, a tip: if you take a fish oil supplement and feel like you are burping up fish, first, make sure it's not expired, and second, try keeping the bottle in the freezer. It works!

Choline

Choline is super necessary during pregnancy, but it's not found in many prenatals—or in the right quantity—so you may want to put it on the list. Found in eggs, organ meat, red meat, and some fish, as well as in plant-based foods like legumes and cruciferous vegetables (though to a smaller extent), choline builds and maintains mama's cell membranes, brain, nervous system, and muscles. It also regulates your metabolism. As far as your baby is concerned, choline is crucial for brain development, preventing neural tube defects, and for placental function.

While you can obtain a decent amount of choline from food, many women's diets fall short, especially if they don't eat eggs. The RDA for pregnancy is four hundred fifty milligrams and five hundred fifty milligrams for breastfeeding. Studies looking at neurodevelopment benefits are using nine hundred milligrams or more, so getting more than the RDA may be a good idea.

Iron

As noted earlier, many women can't tolerate iron in their prenatals because it causes constipation. If that's the case with you, take a prenatal without iron and add in an iron supplement, preferably in the form of iron bisglycinate, as it is better absorbed with fewer side effects, or a desiccated liver supplement.

Vitamin D$_3$

Unless you are able to get thirty minutes or more of midday sun and your levels are in optimal range, you need to take a supplement. (I once heard a saying that if your shadow is taller than you, you're not getting enough vitamin D.)

Chances are good your prenatal does not contain enough D$_3$. Vitamin D is a superstar, reducing the risk of many pregnancy-related complications like preeclampsia, gestational diabetes, and having a low-birth-weight infant. It also bolsters both your and your baby's immune systems and your and your baby's bone and hormone development. This isn't surprising, right? Once upon a time we spent a lot of time outside, and now we spend most of the day behind a computer or in our cars. There are so many connections between nature and our health, and the life-giving aspects of the sun is the brightest one—pun intended.

When looking for a D supplement, do just as you did with your prenatal: look for it in D$_3$ form (not D$_2$), which more closely mimics the variety you get from the sun and is absorbed better. Since it is fat soluble, you ideally want to take it along with a meal or snack that contains some fat, like a handful of nuts or avocado toast. While the RDA for D$_3$ is six hundred IUs, the Endocrine Society says that pregnant women may need between one thousand five hundred and two thousand IUs a day. Some studies even recommend four thousand. I recommend starting with two thousand IUs of D$_3$ per day, which should prevent deficiency, and getting your levels checked after a few months. Supplement accordingly.

Probiotics

Probiotics are healthy, live bacteria, and products that contain them are *everywhere* these days. Kombucha, anyone?

During pregnancy, there are many reasons to add probiotics into your supplement mix, especially since most prenatals don't contain them at all. Maintaining a healthy gut and microbiome is imperative for overall health and especially during pregnancy and nursing. (I'll talk about this more in chapter 4.) If you have a history of antibiotic use, it's even more so, since antibiotics kill both the bad bacteria (like strep) and the beneficial guys. Research shows that the inclusion of probiotic-rich foods and/or supplements, especially in late pregnancy, can reduce a child's risk of developing chronic immune diseases like eczema, dermatitis, food allergies, and asthma. They also play a big part in regulating blood sugar during pregnancy through nursing and beyond.

There are a lot of food sources for probiotics that we'll turn to in the next chapter. In terms of supplements, some brands brands are good refrigerated while others are not, so consult the label on yours. A probiotic should also contain the strains *Lactobacillus rhamnosus*, *Lactobacillus acidophilus,* and *Bifidobacterium*. These can prevent urinary tract infections, gestational diabetes, preeclampsia, and anxiety and depression.

Magnesium

Magnesium deserves a special callout since many people go into pregnancy deficient. If you experience constipation, leg cramps, headaches, or poor sleep—all hallmarks of magnesium deficiency—I recommend supplementing beyond what's in your prenatal.

All magnesium is not created equal. Here are some of your options:

· **Magnesium glycinate:** Derived from glycine, this is the most absorbable form and what I typically use. It helps with anxiety and sleeplessness. Magnesium malate is also well absorbed.

· **Magnesium citrate:** This is magnesium in salt form with citric acid. It can ease constipation and night leg cramps. It can also cause loose stools, so you may need to reduce your dose or take it only a few times a week.

- **Magnesium oxalate and carbonate:** These are cheaper versions of magnesium that won't help pregnant women, and in fact may make you gassy. Avoid them.

- **Epsom salt:** This is your excuse to take a bath or foot soak. Toss one to two cups into your tub. Your skin will sop up all the magnesium in the salt while you achieve peak relaxation (which I know you need).

Regardless of which type you take, magnesium is safe for pregnancy (though if you suffer from kidney disease, you should consult with your doctor first). Start with a lower daily dose (around one hundred milligrams) and slowly build up to three hundred to five hundred milligrams, if needed, while doing the math on what's already in your prenatal. Possible side effects include diarrhea, in which case reduce your dose and chat with your health-care provider. If you continue to feel sick, stop taking magnesium.

SPECIAL CONSIDERATIONS FOR VEGETARIANS AND VEGANS

I understand and value plant-based diets from an environmental, ethical, physical, and emotional standpoint. I don't want to convert anyone or make them feel uncomfortable or judged in their choices. My goal as a dietitian is always to meet clients where they are in terms of nutrition while at the same time providing them with science-backed information so they can make the most informed decisions. While it is entirely possible to have a nutritionally sound pregnancy as a vegan or vegetarian, it's harder because many of the critical vitamins and minerals (including vitamins B_{12} and D, iron, iodine, zinc, and omega-3 DHA) aren't readily available in plant-based foods. Therefore, I can't wholeheartedly recommend a vegetarian or vegan diet during this unique time in your life. But if you decide to stay away from animal protein during pregnancy, consider adding in these supplements:

- **Iron:** This will be one of the more problematic food areas during pregnancy. Iron from a plant-based diet is called nonheme, and it is present in foods like green leafy veggies, such as cooked spinach and kale, and others like beans, lentils, tofu, and pumpkin seeds. Unfortunately, the body only absorbs between 2 and 13 percent of the iron from these foods compared to 25 to 40 percent of the iron from animal-based foods. As such, it is vital to have your iron levels checked before, during (multiple times!), and after pregnancy. Most likely you will have to supplement beyond your typical prenatal vitamin. I've also listed some other suggestions to boost iron intake on page 42.

· **Vitamin B$_{12}$:** I've talked about B$_{12}$ on pages 17, 23, and 31, but it's worth mentioning again. Vegetarians and vegans should consider taking extra B$_{12}$.

· **Choline:** Women who are vegetarian and vegan will most likely not be able to obtain enough from food (as it mostly comes from eggs and organ meats), so think about supplementing or choose a prenatal vitamin that includes choline.

· **Iodine:** Research shows that one quarter of vegetarians and 80 percent of vegans are deficient in iodine, so having enough in your prenatal is key (see the chart on page 34).

· **Omega-3s:** Vegetarians tend to have low levels of EPA and DHA, and vegans have virtually none. Taking an algae-based supplement that contains DHA and EPA (check the labels) is crucial.

· **Zinc:** The zinc found in plant-based diets is less bioavailable than in animal proteins, so be sure your prenatal contains this nutrient.

Finally, if you stick to a vegetarian or vegan diet, make sure your doctor tests your blood every trimester. If you're experiencing uncomfortable side effects or if one of your nutrient levels is out of whack, you can tailor your diet and your supplement regimen accordingly.

HOW TO BOOST YOUR IRON INTAKE

If your iron levels are low or if you become anemic, read this carefully, because there are steps you can take to boost your iron intake. They include the following:

· **Eat red meat or organ meat:** Consume red meat twice a week or eat about three ounces of organ meat (such as liver) per week.

· **Add in vitamin C:** Vitamin C enhances the absorption of iron, so include vitamin-C-rich food when you're eating iron-rich food. For example, cook beef with tomato sauce, marinate chicken in lemon juice, pair salmon and spinach, try a broccoli and cheese baked potato, or whip up a tofu and bell pepper stir-fry.

· **Try cast iron:** Cast-iron skillets have been shown to increase the amount of iron in your food.

· **Supplement:** Iron (in the form of iron bisglycinate) or desiccated liver supplements can help. Make sure to separate your iron supplement from any calcium supplement (or any prenatal multivitamin containing calcium) by at least two to three hours, as the two nutrients compete for absorption.

· **Keep testing:** Have your blood work done again a few months after you're diagnosed with low iron or anemia (and have followed these steps). You may be pleasantly surprised to see that your levels have gone up to within a normal range.

THE BOTTOM LINE

At the end of the day—and with all you have to think about during pregnancy—I'd love for you to not have to worry about what supplements you take. I hope they can become a seamless and automatic part of your daily routine. That being said, doing a little work up front, getting your blood tested, seeing what your levels are, and finding the right brands and quantities that suit your needs will make things so much easier. I know it's hard; the first trimester can be rough, and pill popping is the last thing on your mind. But just know that the decisions and actions you take right now will have a significant effect. Trust me, you'll be happy you took the time.

CHAPTER 3

FOODS TO
NOURISH AND PROTECT MOM

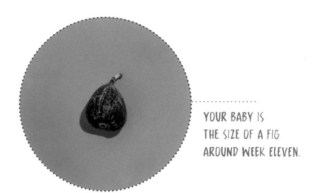

YOUR BABY IS
THE SIZE OF A FIG
AROUND WEEK ELEVEN.

You've got the prenatal, you've done the blood work, and you've picked up any additional supplements you may need. Great. Now we can focus on what we're all here to talk about: *food*. Remember this: nothing is better for you and your baby than real, whole, healthy food. Food is the fuel that will get you through the tough periods, nurture you and baby, and make everything—including the postpartum months—a lot easier.

I know how yucky you can feel during the first trimester and that food is most likely the last thing on your mind. In fact, maybe you're going out of your way to avoid it altogether. We will push through to start your pregnancy on the right foot with foods rich in key nutrients that support you and your baby. The more you consume them, the more your body will crave them over time. If you put in this little bit of effort now, it will pay big dividends later.

PROTEIN

Protein is your main priority. Proteins are the building blocks of life, and recent research shows that your protein needs increase throughout pregnancy (so you will require more in your third trimester than your first). While women in the first trimester should get between seventy-five and one hundred grams a day, in the third trimester, it jumps up to a minimum of one hundred grams a day. Proteins (including collagen and amino acids, like glycine) stabilize your blood sugar, regulate your pH, transport nutrients, help increase your blood supply, and build tissues and muscles. They also promote every aspect of your baby's development, growth, and metabolism—from the reproductive system to their tiny muscles. If you are constantly hungry and feel especially low in energy, it could be a sign you need to up your protein intake.

There is a ton of conflicting information about whether plant- or animal-based protein is better for health, since plants are richer in some dietary components, and animal sources are richer in others. You can make a case for both, so I advise you to look for a combination of animal- and plant-based proteins. Plant-based proteins deliver fiber, folate, and vitamin C. However, I believe that animal proteins, which provide key nutrients like iron, B_{12}, zinc, choline, and DHA (and which help mama stay healthy and baby develop), are necessary during pregnancy and postpartum.

The goal is to include a protein with every meal and snack—and trust me, if you weren't a snacker before, you will need to be one now. Quality counts too. When possible, aim for meat from grass-fed or pasture-raised animals, which contain higher levels of omega-3s, beta-carotene, and vitamin E, among other nutrients, than conventionally raised animals.

If proteins make you sick to your stomach, do not stress. Do the best you can. You don't need to eat a gigantic meal at every sitting; a little bit here and there does wonders. Remember, you crave what you eat, so getting in a bite or two will make you want it more once your pregnancy progresses and you start to feel better.

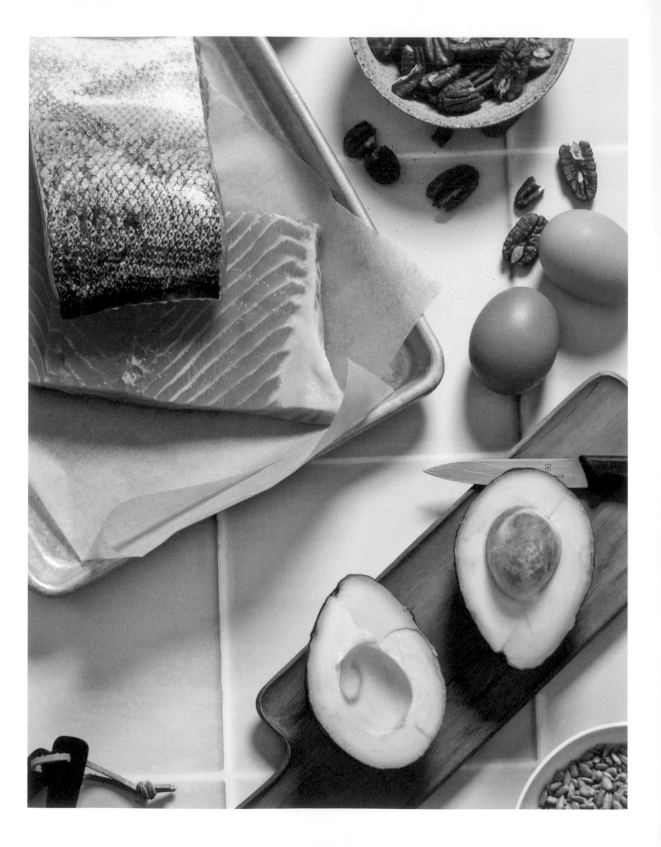

Rich protein sources include the following:

· **Eggs:** Ideally from pasture-raised birds and in any form you crave. Eggs are one of the best sources of choline except for organ meats, like liver.

· **Red meat:** Beef, lamb, and game meat like bison or venison, ideally from pasture-raised animals.

· **Fish and shellfish:** Preferably wild caught.

· **Poultry:** Ideally from pasture-raised animals.

· **Dairy:** Milk, pasteurized cheese, cottage cheese, and yogurt (plain, full fat, and pasteurized), ideally from grass-fed or pasture-raised animals.

· **Bone broth**

· **Lentils, beans, nuts/seeds, nut and seed butter, peas, and tofu**

BONE BROTH FOR THE WIN

It's trendy, it's everywhere, and it's beloved by celebrity chefs and grandmas alike. The hype exists for a reason. Bones are one of the most nutritious parts of an animal, and the vitamins and minerals in bone broth (like iron; copper; zinc; calcium; phosphorus; magnesium; vitamins A, C, K; and all the B vitamins) can support bone health and your immune system, as well as aid with postpartum healing. Your body metabolizes liquids quickly, so every time you sip bone broth, it's like you're downing a prenatal vitamin, and it can feel especially nourishing and hydrating.

Making bone broth is simple (see page 247). You can also order it online or buy it from a store; if you choose a reputable brand that's preferably made from bones of organic, grass-fed animals, it's just as good as making it at home, and you'll save time (although it will cost you more than making it yourself). Sip it like tea or use it as a base for soups, stir-fries, quinoa, and rice. Just swap water with the same amount of bone broth in any recipe. Aim for one to two cups a day.

You can freeze bone broth for up to six months, so if you're game to play home chef, then you can make a huge batch to dole out over the next few months. I consumed a lot of bone broth when I was pregnant and postpartum, especially in the first trimester when not many foods appealed. My kids love it too, and I find it's really healing when they are sick. It's also a terrific source of nutrition when you or your kids are nauseated and can't keep much else down.

What if you're a vegetarian or vegan? While vegetable-based broths have their own pluses, they don't have the same nutritional benefits. Bones contain much more protein than any vegetable, and plants don't have collagen. Again, though, any form of nutrition is better than none, so enjoy vegetable broth if that's what you have. No matter what, it will keep you hydrated and will give you micronutrients from those good veggies.

EATING ORGAN MEATS DURING PREGNANCY

Bear with me. While organ meats like liver are foreign to many of us or remind us of unpleasant meals at grandma's house, gram for gram, liver provides more nutrients than any other food. Yup, liver is extremely nutrient dense and is particularly rich in iron, choline (only eggs contain as much), and vitamin B_{12}, folate, and vitamin A. You know by now that these are all extremely important in pregnancy.

A little liver goes a long way, so consuming three to six ounces a week gives a lot of bang for your buck. Liver is especially great for those who are anemic and can't tolerate iron supplements, because it gives you a ton of absorbable heme iron. Not only that, liver is relatively inexpensive compared to other cuts of meat, plus you're typically not purchasing a large amount.

Still not convinced? How about if I tell you that liver can be really tasty, especially if you mix it in with meatloaf, meatballs, or chili? Still not there? That's fine. You can still get these key nutrients from other foods.

FOOD MYTH: DAIRY

Dairy is a controversial topic. Some people claim that it is inflammatory and should be avoided, while others preach its benefits and want you to get in multiple servings a day (hello, food pyramid!), especially if you're pregnant.

My answer is . . . it depends. It depends on how you react to dairy or if you have a specific reason that consuming it wouldn't be good for your body. People with GI issues (gas, bloating, constipation, diarrhea, inflammatory bowel disease [IBD], acid reflux) may feel a whole lot better without dairy. Same for folks with skin issues like eczema or inflammatory conditions like psoriasis, celiac disease, and Hashimoto's thyroiditis. Congestion is related to inflammation, so if you're pregnant and going through tissue boxes daily, try eliminating dairy for two to three weeks and see if your symptoms improve. In fact, it's great to test and trial if you sense dairy might be an issue for you. A lot of people can consume dairy in smaller amounts (meaning smaller portions or a few times a week instead of daily) without any issues, so you can reintroduce it slowly to gauge. Other people tolerate dairy products from sheep or goats (like feta or Manchego cheese or pasteurized goat's milk) better than foods made from cow's milk. I always feel that knowing what doesn't make you feel good puts you in the driver's seat, so you can make the decision for yourself.

If you can tolerate any dairy with no problems, then, by all means, go for it. Dairy is a wonderful source of nutrition for pregnant women (containing calcium; fat-soluble vitamins A, D, E, and K; potassium; iodine; and easy-to-consume protein and fat). You should also include fermented dairy like kefir, yogurt, and cottage cheese, which may feel okay even if you've had issues with dairy before. Some people develop lactose intolerance in pregnancy, and some people with lactose intolerance have it *reversed* while pregnant (mine reversed, and it was amazing while it lasted). Choose sources that are pasteurized, and that are full-fat and grass-fed when possible.

WHAT IF YOU DON'T CONSUME DAIRY?

Perhaps one of the most common questions I receive is how to get enough calcium, especially if you can't or don't eat dairy. It's no wonder: calcium is crucial, especially starting in the second trimester, when the mother's body absorbs and metabolizes two to three times more calcium than it did pre-pregnancy. Fortunately and unfortunately, if a mother-to-be doesn't get enough calcium to supply her baby's bones, her body will start taking it from *her* bones. That's why building up stores *pronto* is paramount.

But here is the thing: calcium isn't the only mineral in town that helps with bone formation. It works synergistically with vitamin D, vitamin K, and magnesium to build strong bones and assist in numerous metabolic processes. While foods rich in these vitamins and minerals may not be enough to give your baby's teeth and bones what they need, you don't have to rely on dairy alone. If you don't or can't consume dairy, certain nondairy calcium sources I mention below, as well as foods rich in vitamin D, vitamin K, and magnesium, should ensure your requirements are met. Try to get in at least one or two of these nondairy sources a day and consume plenty of fat to help absorb vitamins D and K, which are fat soluble.

Calcium-rich nondairy foods include the following:

· Canned fish like salmon and sardines. They're not for everyone (I am personally not a sardine fan), but the bones of these tiny fish are a gold mine of calcium. Just pop a few on your sandwich or salad.

- Chia seeds
- Green veggies like kale, bok choy, broccoli, mustard greens, and spinach. A note on spinach: it is high in calcium, but it also contains oxalates, which interfere with calcium absorption. However, if you cook spinach it helps to break down the oxalates.
- Almonds
- Tofu
- Sesame seeds, including tahini
- Bone broth made from grass-fed bones
- Fortified plant-based milk (just be sure to shake the container before serving)

FAT

Fat is your second priority. Say it with me: fat is your friend. Take a spin around the kitchen, and toss (or give away) low-fat anything. Fat just makes things better by being delicious and nourishing to mama and baby. Fats are also crucial for the absorption of fat-soluble vitamins like vitamins A, D, E, and K. You don't want that prenatal you take every day to go to waste! Fats play a central role in hormone production, and hormones are working in overdrive right now. Finally, fats are filled with essential fatty acids like omega-3s.

Aim to include at least one fat source per meal. Healthy fats come in different types, and they include the following:

- **Monounsaturated fats:** Sources include avocados, olives, certain nuts (almonds, cashews, macadamia nuts, and pecans), seeds like pumpkin and sesame, extra-virgin olive oil, and avocado oil.

- **Polyunsaturated fats:** Found in fish (salmon, trout, anchovies, and sardines), walnuts, plant-based oils, and seeds (flax and chia).

- **Omega-3s:** As discussed in the previous chapter, omega-3s are polyunsaturated fats that support brain development and reduce inflammation. They are DHA, EPA, and ALA.

- **Saturated fats:** Coconut (coconut oil and plain coconut yogurt), dairy such as full-fat yogurt, cottage cheese, and cheese, and grass-fed animal proteins.

WATCH OUT: VEGETABLE OILS

One type of fat to *limit* is omega-6, which is found in seed oils, including canola, soy, peanut, cottonseed, and safflower (yes, a peanut is a legume and seed, despite its name). These seed oils are also known as vegetable oils, and while that may sound healthy, when they're heated or exposed to air, they become unstable. That creates free radicals that can damage your cells and inhibit DNA synthesis.

Don't cook with them, and read your labels. You'd be surprised by how ubiquitous they are. A little bit won't hurt you, so as with everything else, don't get obsessed about skipping out on your favorite restaurant or anything else that brings you joy, but proceed with caution.

Instead, go with one of these options:

- **Olive oil:** It's full of protective antioxidants that can promote brain development. Even at high temperatures and when exposed to air, it's the oil least likely to create free radicals. Choose extra-virgin, and drizzle it on bread, use it in salad dressings, and cook with it—it's delicious subbed in most recipes, even desserts.

- **Avocado oil:** Avocado oil helps you absorb antioxidants, and I love it for cooking at extra-high temperatures.

- **Coconut oil:** Coconut oil is rich in medium-chain fatty acids (MCFAs), which can help provide a quick boost of energy. It's also a great plant-based alternative to butter and is wonderful in baked goods, stir-fries, and curries.

- **Flaxseed oil:** Rich in omega-3s, flaxseed is not a cooking oil but is wonderful in salad dressing, smoothies, and yogurt.

- **Ghee (clarified butter):** This one is technically not an oil, but it's a go-to for cooking at high temperatures. It is a dairy product, but the dairy solids have been removed, and it doesn't contain casein and lactose. Some people with dairy sensitivities find that they can tolerate ghee just fine.

- **Butter:** There is nothing wrong with good old-fashioned butter! It is rich in vitamins and minerals, including vitamins A, D, E, K. Although also technically not an oil, you can definitely bring butter back into your cooking rotation.

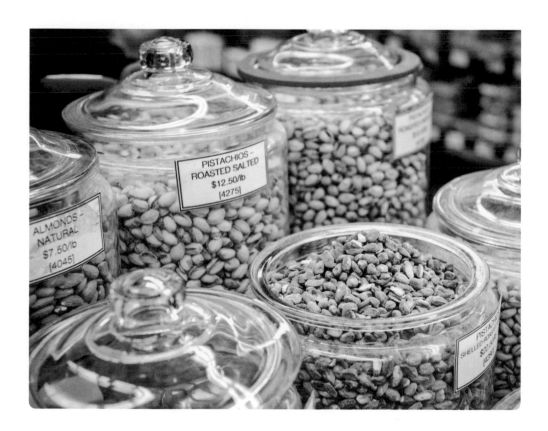

VEGETABLES

This one is a no-brainer, but I have to say it anyway. Veggies should *always* be the stars on your plate, and they have a lot of added benefits during pregnancy. All vegetables contain antioxidants, vitamins, and minerals that support your gut microbiome and help with digestion. Green veggies are especially rich in folate—central to fetal growth—and fiber, which keeps you regular (I'll get into that later). You should include the full rainbow of vegetables in your meals, as most are chock-full of vitamin C (which helps with the absorption of iron), vitamin K, vitamin A, calcium, folate, magnesium, and potassium.

Eat vegetables however you like, whether raw (as long they are as well washed) or cooked. I also love fermented or pickled vegetables like sauerkraut, kimchi, cucumbers, beets, radishes, and carrots, which are rich sources of probiotics that support the gut and immune system. A fun game is to see how many colors you can incorporate into a day's meals—the more, the better. **The goal is to make half your plate veggies (roughly two fistfuls or two cups) at lunch and dinner.**

Maybe vegetables hold no appeal for you at the moment, and that is normal and okay. In those first few months of my pregnancies, I ate a limited quantity of vegetables. I wanted them raw, cold, and a bit on the sour side, so I could tolerate only crunchy iceberg or romaine lettuce, purple cabbage with olive oil and salt, an Asian-inspired slaw, and a cucumber salad that I made every day. If you're experiencing morning sickness, try including a little portion of vegetables on your plate—just a bite or two—and once your nausea subsides, you will find yourself wanting more.

For some of the more "tolerable" veggie recipes, check out the recipes starting on page 221, as well as some ways to sneak them in—in muffins, waffles, sauces (e.g., pesto), and smoothies. Now that I'm a mom, I'm an expert sneaky veggie chef.

FRUITS

Fruit is often a major craving for pregnant women. It was for me. I can't tell you how many oranges I consumed in the earlier months, and I could not get enough watermelon at the end of my pregnancy. It's no wonder: fruit is hydrating and refreshing, and you're often dehydrated during pregnancy. I especially love frozen grapes—they're nature's candy and can provide much-needed relief for anyone having a summer baby.

Each type of fruit provides its own set of benefits, so aim for variety. For example, pineapple is rich in an enzyme mixture called bromelain that aids digestion; apples contain antioxidants, which assist with lung development (both yours and your baby's); and berries are full of vitamin C, which enhances iron absorption, and fiber, which keeps you regular.

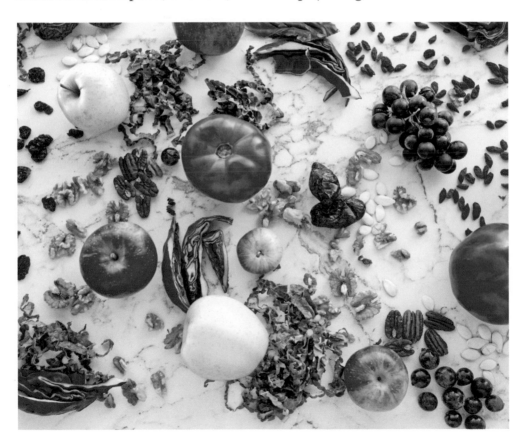

Eating pineapple will not cause you to miscarry or go into early labor. While bromelain can soften the cervix (so supplements are not recommended for pregnant women), the amount of bromelain present in a few servings of pineapple is not enough to cause any issues.

For those who need to be cautious with blood sugar, try to keep to one cup of cut-up fruit (or one handheld fruit, e.g., an apple or a pear) at once and pair it with a protein like nuts, nut butter, full-fat yogurt, or cottage cheese, which will prevent your sugar from spiking.

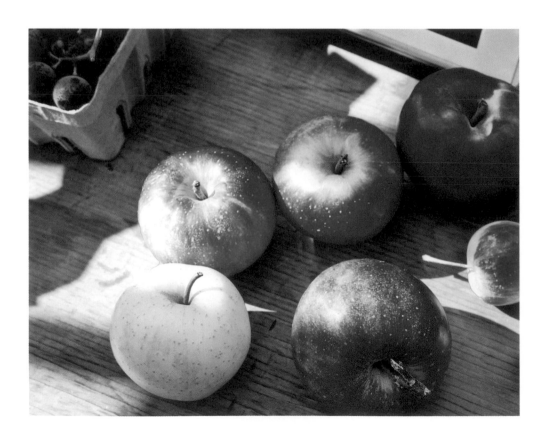

CARBOHYDRATES

Whether or not you were into carbs before, you will be now. In fact, carbs—that is, starches and grains—may be all you want in those first few months. I lived on sourdough bread and grass-fed butter, which is still a comfort combo for me. The key is to aim for healthier forms, called complex carbohydrates. These include oats, sweet potatoes (or any potatoes), winter squashes (butternut, acorn, etc.), and whole grains like farro and buckwheat. When you do need that carb fix, choose foods and products that are made with minimal ingredients and won't lead to a major blood sugar spike and subsequent crash—so think whole-grain bread with peanut butter rather than a stack of pancakes. That being said, if you are craving that bowl of white rice or something similar, pair it with a healthy protein so that your blood sugar doesn't crash as fast; that alone is a positive step toward nourishing your body.

Know that there is a wide range of ways pregnant women respond to carbs. You don't have to include them with every meal. Some do better with fewer carbs, while others thrive with more. Experiment with what works for you. When you do include them, **your goal is to fill a quarter of your plate with complex carbs (the remainder should be protein, fats, and vegetables/fruits).** Simply being aware of this balance at each meal is a huge win.

A NOTE ON PORTIONS

As you may notice, I'm not strict with recommended portions and often don't even provide them. The ideal portion varies from person to person based on size, activity level, age, and more. Your needs will shift at different stages in your pregnancy, and even day to day. For example, you will likely need more carbs in the first trimester and more protein in your third trimester. I will say this: if for whatever reason you have a health concern, like gestational diabetes or too much or too little weight gain (based on an evaluation from your provider) you may benefit from working with a registered dietitian to make a plan geared specifically to you.

WHY QUALITY MATTERS

Being pregnant is overwhelming (that's an understatement!), and choosing the healthiest alternatives for yourself and your baby can be hard. But if there is one thing that you should take away from this book, it's that quality *does* matter. Now, I've said again and again—do your best and don't let the perfect be the enemy of the good. But quality is the one area where if you can stretch and take that extra step, do it. Your efforts and the expense will pay significant dividends down the line.

What does quality mean? It means choosing the least processed foods you can find—items that are organic, local (when possible), grass-fed, pasture-raised, pole-caught, etc. There is clear, demonstrable proof that these foods are healthier, safer, and often tastier than their counterparts. Organic foods pack in better nutrition, and organically grown fruits, grains, and vegetables contain higher levels of antioxidants. Grass-fed livestock contains higher levels of vitamin E and omega-3 fatty acids. You'll spend more on organic produce and grass-fed meat, but as far as nutrition goes, you get more bang for your buck.

What's even more significant is that organic foods don't carry as many of the chemicals you *do not* want in your body on a good day, let alone when there is a tiny human living inside you. For instance, a 2014 study showed that organic foods contain 48 percent less cadmium—a toxic metal that is categorized as a class 1 carcinogen—than conventionally grown foods. Pregnant women are more vulnerable to toxins than nonpregnant women, and studies show that expectant mothers exposed to certain environmental toxins have higher rates of preeclampsia and gestational diabetes. These toxins can be transferred to babies through the placenta and breast milk—in fact, studies have found that up to two hundred kinds of industrial chemicals and pollutants can be found in umbilical cord blood.

If you're feeling overwhelmed, take a deep breath. Awareness is half the battle, and making small changes is better than doing nothing at all. I certainly don't buy organic products all the time—and I've written two books with *organic* in their titles. Nor do I think organic means "perfect." Heck, even organic methods do use some forms of pesticides.

Here's how you identify foods for quality:

- **Eggs:** Purchase pasture-raised eggs, because the hens live outside, with access to grass and bugs and other foods they love. This leads to higher levels of protein, vitamin E, and omega-3 fats. If you can't find (or afford) pasture-raised eggs, choose organic (meaning that the hens were fed organic grain). If you can't buy organic, try free-range (meaning that they were allowed to roam around a barn, though they may have been packed in tightly). "Raised without antibiotics or hormones" means nothing; in the US, it's against the law to give chickens antibiotics or hormones, so that is literally the bare minimum you can expect. Finally, know that it's better to eat an egg than none at all, so purchase and consume whatever you can.

- **Dairy:** Aim to buy grass-fed dairy, because that means it comes from cows that have grazed on grass, wheat, and flowers in a pasture. Their milk contains more omega-3s. If you can't buy or afford grass-fed, try organic, which means it's hormone- and contaminant-free, and the cows eat a diet that consists of at least 30 percent grass.

- **Meat:** Look for grass-fed meat, which contains more omega-3s, vitamin E, and beta-carotene and less pesticide residue. It comes from happier cows that have been treated humanely. If you can't buy grass-fed, the next best is organic. Although the meat is likely not from grass-fed cows (unless indicated), it won't be from cows that were fed genetically modified, pesticide-filled soy or corn. Ideally, get to know the source; if you're at a farmers market, for example, ask the farmer about their practices. Their products might not be certified organic, for example, but they may use similar or even better techniques.

- **Seafood:** The USDA doesn't classify seafood as "organic" or "conventional." However, wild-caught seafood will likely contain more nutrients and fewer toxins than farm-raised seafood. Fish is a loaded topic during pregnancy because of concerns about mercury and other toxins. I'll talk about that later in this chapter.

- **Produce:** Local produce is fresher, and it supports your community. However, getting certified organic is expensive, and many local farms use organic practices but can't afford the certification. As with meat and dairy, when in doubt, ask the farmer. If you don't have access to or can't afford local or organic, focus on the Dirty Dozen list (see below) to prioritize your fruits and veggies. If there is one food you are eating daily, think about investing in organic for that item.

Whatever you choose, enjoy what you're eating and aim for whole foods, even if they aren't organic. Eating a conventionally grown apple is still much better than avoiding apples, and eating a non-pasture-raised egg is still better than skipping eggs. Below is a useful list created by the Environmental Working Group (EWG), a nonprofit environmental advocacy group that releases the "Dirty Dozen" and the "Clean Fifteen" lists every year, highlighting the conventionally grown fruits and vegetables that are as good as organic, and which ones to avoid.

THE DIRTY DOZEN AND THE CLEAN FIFTEEN

THE DIRTY DOZEN

These are the top twelve fruits and vegetables most affected by agricultural pesticides, so try as hard as you can to purchase the organic varieties: (1) strawberries, (2) spinach, (3) kale, collard, and mustard greens, (4) peaches, (5) pears, (6) nectarines, (7) apples, (8) grapes, (9) bell and hot peppers, (10) cherries, (11) blueberries, and (12) green beans.

THE CLEAN FIFTEEN

These fifteen fruits and vegetables are less affected by pesticides, so this is a good place to save your money: (1) avocados, (2) sweet corn, (3) pineapple, (4) onions, (5) papaya, (6) sweet peas (frozen), (7) asparagus, (8) honeydew melon, (9) kiwi, (10) cabbage, (11) mushrooms, (12) mangoes, (13) sweet potatoes, (14) watermelon, and (15) carrots.

THE IMPORTANCE OF HYDRATION

You've heard it a million times, most likely from a parent or a coach. Guess what? You're now going to hear it from me. DRINK MORE WATER.

Everyone knows that staying hydrated is one of the easiest things you can do to be healthy, but it should be at the top of your to-do list when you're expecting. Let me put my lab coat on for a second. When your baby is growing, your blood volume also increases—by as much as 50 percent! What is blood made of? Yep, that's right, water—so this is part of why you may feel like you are constantly thirsty. Water replenishes your amniotic fluid, aids in circulation (preventing leg cramps), regulates body temperature, and alleviates and prevents constipation and swollen limbs. Finally, adequate hydration helps prevent preterm labor.

You're going to need twelve cups of water per day. That's about one hundred ounces for those keeping track. Now, that's a lot of water, but it includes the water found in the foods you eat, so pick lots of juicy fruits and vegetables and you'll be well on your way. You should still get about half to three quarters of your water the old-fashioned way, so find a glass or stainless-steel water bottle and make it your best friend.

Oh, and one other thing, before you ask—no, coffee doesn't count.

HYDRATION HANG-UPS

One hundred ounces of water a day is a lot, and it can get, well, boring. It's often hard to drink water when you're suffering from morning sickness as well. To keep things interesting (and to keep you hydrated when the thought of anything in your stomach makes you ill), try the following:

· **Add citrus**: Toss a few lemon, lime, or orange wedges into your glass. You'll get a dose of vitamin C and fiber *and* level up the taste, and the smell of citrus can calm an unsettled stomach. I was a huge fan of unwinding at night with a cup of warm water and lemon before bed.

- **Hydrate early:** Drink eight ounces of water first thing in the morning. If you're feeling nauseated, sip rather than chug, and eat a few bites of food first.

- **Adjust the temperature:** Try drinking really cold water rather than room temperature. Or try a warm cup of water with honey and lemon, which might soothe your belly.

- **Think about timing:** Drink a glass of water before every meal, which can make food more palatable.

- **Try other fluids:** If you can't stomach water, try tea, coconut water, or smoothies and bone broth, all of which are just as hydrating.

- **Freeze it:** Grab a silicone ice tray, add coconut water and fresh fruit, pop it in the freezer, and voilà. Fruity ice cubes are delicious in seltzer or plain old water.

- **Try electrolyte packets:** A handful of brands make electrolyte drink packets without added sugar or preservatives. Start with half a packet and then build up to one a day.

- **Imagine yourself at the beach:** Coconut water is refreshing, and it also provides potassium, a vital electrolyte. I recommend drinking one cup with a sprinkle of sea salt for extra sodium.

- **Hydrate with watermelon:** Watermelon is 92 percent water. Freeze it, blend up a watermelon slushie (which can then be frozen into ice pops), or make a watermelon salad with feta, olive oil, flaky sea salt, and fresh mint or basil. Or, make it easy on yourself: eat plain old watermelon cut (or munched) from the rind.

- **Try herbs:** Toss basil or fresh mint leaves with sliced cucumber. Cucumbers contain vitamin C and caffeic acid, which prevent water retention and reduce swelling. See page 271 for my favorite cucumber herb ice pop recipe.

- **Add chia seeds:** Mix two tablespoons of chia seeds with half a cup of water, milk (dairy or nondairy), coconut water, or watermelon water. Chia seeds expand to ten times their size in liquid and thicken quickly into a jellylike consistency. See page 198 for a yummy chia jam recipe.

You can have too much of a good thing. If you're still thirsty after you've had your daily one hundred ounces, that could mean you need more electrolytes. You can supplement through add-ins like electrolyte powders or coconut water, which will replenish the stuff that keeps you hydrated and energized rather than flush it out.

WHAT ABOUT ELECTROLYTES?

Electrolytes are essential minerals that dissolve in fluid and carry a small—but important—electric charge. They include sodium, potassium, chloride, calcium, and magnesium, and they take part in everything from your heart beating normally to preventing cramps.

Because your blood volume increases so much during pregnancy, your electrolyte needs do too. Salt often gets a bad rap, but it is incredibly important to the normal functions of your body, like moving nutrients into and waste out of your cells, facilitating muscle contractions, and regulating nervous system function. Not all salt is made the same, though; the salt in processed food and your basic table salt are different from unrefined sea salt, which contains trace minerals. Choose mineral-rich sea salt and salt your own food (you're much more likely to eat an appropriate amount when you cook at home rather than getting takeout or heating up a frozen dinner).

If you feel cramps, headaches, leg cramps, swelling, tiredness, or generally feel off, add an electrolyte packet into your water or smoothie, mix a pinch of sea salt into coconut water or watermelon water, or make your own electrolyte mix (see page 156.)

The next question I usually get is, What kind of water? Sparkling, mineral, flat, tap? What about water fortified with electrolytes? Is bottled okay? Here's the deal: Bubbles are fine, but they can lead to acid reflux and indigestion, especially during pregnancy, so check out your body's reaction after having a glass. As for bottled versus tap, I suggest getting a water purifier for your home—either a pitcher version or one you can easily install under your sink—and filling up your water bottle. Bottled water isn't terrible, but so much of it comes from municipal sources anyway (meaning it's tap water dressed up fancy), and it's in plastic, which can leach nasty stuff *and* act as an endocrine disruptor in your body. (I'll talk more about plastics and toxins in chapter 4.) Of course, a bottle of water in a pinch is not a big deal, and I'd rather you be hydrated than not, but aim to get in the habit of bringing your water bottle with you wherever you go.

FIGHT THE BLECH!

The first trimester usually means morning sickness, nausea, and bloating—delightful. If you're not experiencing the terrible three, don't worry; it doesn't mean anything for the health of your baby. Give yourself a pat on the back, pass go, collect a yummy meal, and head to the next section. For the rest of you, you're with me.

Every pregnancy is different, even for the same person. Still, roughly 75 percent of pregnant women spend much of their first trimester (or beyond) with nausea and bouts of vomiting. Morning sickness can strike at any time of day, and it may come on quickly and knock you out for a while. It most certainly is not the puke and rally that's portrayed in the movies, and it will most likely last the entirety of your first trimester.

Luckily, there are things you can do to manage your symptoms. First, identify what is causing your nausea. One theory is that morning sickness springs from low blood sugar and hormonal spikes (specifically hCG and estrogen) or from micronutrient deficiencies, especially B_6 and zinc. For others, it might be a sign of acid reflux. There's not much you can do about your pregnancy hormones, so we'll do our best to manage that icky feeling through food. Talk to your doctor about how you are feeling, especially if you are unable to keep anything down. Be sure you're hydrated and receiving sufficient nutrition, and your provider may be able to prescribe medication to help. If you still feel like you're not getting enough nutrition through food—or if you're living on a diet of crackers and coconut—it's okay. Your baby pulls from your nutrient stores, which you have built up over the course of your life.

Below are some methods that should be useful. Having said that, I have worked with women who followed these recommendations and still experienced some morning sickness, so if that's you, know you're not alone.

- **Eat to balance blood sugar:** In terms of satiating hunger and balancing blood sugar, whatever your existing system is most likely won't fly in pregnancy, especially during these early weeks. Aim to include protein and a fat with every meal and snack. Even getting in a few bites of protein before bedtime will make a big impact on your blood sugar and how you feel the next morning. It's equally important to include protein for breakfast, as your body will be more reactive to sugar and carbs on an empty stomach. Even if you aren't hungry or have never been a breakfast person, try to eat a little something. Add nut butter, avocado, or cheese to toast and sprinkle on seeds like chia, ground flax, pumpkin, or hemp, or stir them into oatmeal. You will likely notice you begin to feel hungry in the morning (which is a good thing; your body is doing its job) and hopefully less nauseated. I will talk more about blood sugar in chapter 6.

- **Snack smart:** Instead of reaching for plain crackers, include a fat/protein option like hummus, guacamole, or cheese. Think of your snacks like mini meals in terms of getting the food groups on your plate, and don't worry if you feel the need to eat five or six times during the day (around every two to three hours). This may be a sign that your blood sugar is dipping. Not eating often enough can also increase acid reflux symptoms and nausea.

- **Tackle acid reflux:** When I was pregnant with my daughter, much of my morning sickness was due to acid reflux. Before I figured that out, I thought that a fizzy drink would calm things down, but it made it worse. If the problem is acid reflux, be mindful of triggers like carbonated drinks, alliums such as garlic and onions (leeks and shallots are often more easily tolerated), chocolate, tomatoes or tomato sauce, citrus, and coffee. If you are dying for that cup of coffee, aim to drink it after food or go for a cold brew, which is less acidic. Maintain a balance between not eating too much at one time and not allowing yourself to get too hungry. Keep snacks on hand.

- **Sip slowly:** Sip water throughout the day rather than downing a lot at once. I can't stress this enough: even when you feel sick, drink as much water as you can. Space it out over the course of the day if you need to. Include electrolytes like coconut water plus sea salt, half to a whole packet of an electrolyte mix, or even sip on some bone broth.

- **Smells:** Pay attention to smells that are off-putting and toss 'em. I could not stand coconut *anything* during pregnancy (except coconut-based ice cream—pregnancy is weird!). You may need to call on a member of your support team, whether that's a partner, friend, parent, etc., to help out at mealtime. My husband and I have always shared cooking duties, but I couldn't go near the kitchen during those first few months. Like me, you may need to ask your partner to cook for you until you're back on your feet (point them to page 187 for the recipes!).

- **B vitamins:** Add a B_6 supplement. B_6 is in your prenatal vitamin, but at lower levels than you may need. Roughly ten to twenty milligrams one to two times a day has been shown to provide relief.

- **Ginger:** Whether it's in tea, in a gummy, or pickled, ginger is a great (and clinically proven) way to reduce nausea.

- **Go for the cold:** Frozen fruits like grapes, cherries, and mango were favorites of mine when I had morning sickness. The colder, the better.

- **Sour foods:** It seems counterintuitive, but sour foods can reduce nausea. Add a few lemon slices to your water. Some people also swear by keeping freshly cut lemons to sniff or lick when times get tough.

- **Non-food-related tips:** While getting out of bed might be the last thing you want to do, light exercise (like a walk) can be a big help. Motion sickness bracelets are also popular. Try to sleep in a cool room at night, because overheating can increase nausea. Stress can also aggravate

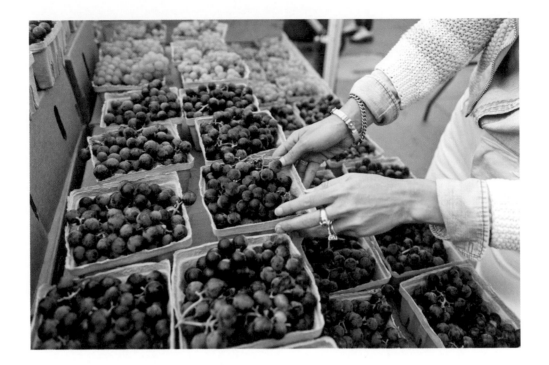

morning sickness, and studies have found that increased cortisol (the stress hormone) contributes to blood sugar issues; look into stress-reduction techniques, like exercise, deep breathing, and acupuncture. I had fantastic results with acupuncture in both of my pregnancies.

THE P WORD

I have to warn you, poop is a favorite topic of mine. It is a key part of anyone's nutrition journey and also a major factor in pregnancy. During the first trimester, you may feel like you have to poop all the time, but you may not be able to. Constipation is a huge bummer, no way around it—but there are ways to make it better.

Let's talk about the causes so we can talk about the solutions. During the first trimester (especially the second and third month), progesterone levels rise dramatically, and that relaxes your muscles, including the intestines. As your intestines work slower, digestion slows too, and that can lead to constipation.

Also, many people have issues when their prenatal contains iron and often find relief by switching to one without. You'll just have to get your iron a different way, either through food or as a separate supplement. Finally, a lot of women find it hard to eat fiber-rich foods in the first trimester, so their intake goes down—bam, constipation.

It may not surprise you that my number one piece of advice is to DRINK MORE WATER. If you only get those one hundred ounces in, things will improve. Adequate hydration allows the intestines to operate optimally, and on the flip side, dehydration can lead to hard, slow-moving stools.

Next—fiber, specifically of the insoluble variety. Your best sources are vegetables (especially leafy greens like kale, Swiss chard, and spinach), fruits (berries in particular), beans, and seeds like flax and chia (just make sure the flaxseed is ground, otherwise it will go right through you). Aim to get in thirty grams of fiber a day (versus twenty-five grams when you're not pregnant). When you add extra fiber into your diet, do it slowly; increasing it too quickly can cause gas and bloating. If you're feeling sick, it may be hard to eat fiber, so just do your best. A little is better than nothing.

FIBER FUELED

Confused about which foods contain fiber? This chart shows some easy sources of fiber for your snacks and meals. You don't need to count grams (it's just not worth it), but if you are having trouble going to the bathroom, do what you can to get up to thirty grams by eating a combination of the following foods.

FOOD SOURCE	SERVING SIZE	TOTAL FIBER (G)
Split peas, cooked	1 cup	16
Lentils	1 cup	15.5
Black beans, boiled	1 cup	15
White beans	½ cup	9.5
Green peas, cooked	1 cup	9
Raspberries	1 cup	8
Barley, pearled, cooked	1 cup	6
Pear	1 medium	5.5
Psyllium husk	1 tablespoon	5
Broccoli, cooked	1 cup	5
Turnip greens, cooked	1 cup	5
Quinoa, cooked	1 cup	5
Oatmeal, cooked	1 cup	5
Avocado	½ cup	5
Collard greens, cooked	1 cup	5
Spinach, cooked	1 cup	4.5
Apple, with skin	1 medium	4.5
Chia seeds	1 tablespoon	4
Brussels sprouts, cooked	1 cup	4
Potato with skin, baked	1 medium	4
Ground flaxseed	1 tablespoon	3
Pistachios	1 ounce	3

Now for the pièce de résistance: fat. I've already talked about how clutch fat is in pregnancy, and when it comes to avoiding constipation, fat lubricates your intestines, making everything go more smoothly.

If you've tried all of the above, and it's just not helping, it's time for extra support (and I don't mean laxatives). Incorporate more magnesium into your diet. Leafy greens are a fantastic way to get magnesium, but if you can't stand the thought of roughage, add kale, spinach, or Swiss chard to a smoothie. Nuts and seeds are also high in magnesium, so snack on almonds, Brazil nuts, and squash and pumpkin seeds, or bake them into a healthy treat.

You can also add a magnesium citrate or glycinate supplement, which I discussed in the previous chapter. Start with the lower end of the recommended amount; if you don't have problems, you can increase the dosage to a max of five hundred milligrams. But if you have any cramping or loose stools, then bring it back down or take it only a few times a week.

YES, NO, AND SOMETIMES FOODS

There is *so* much misinformation, conjecture, and fear around "forbidden" foods. Eat this, don't eat that; if you come across a sushi bar, quickly cross the street; and make sure all your meat is cooked to the point where you can't even chew it.

I'll try to make it simple. There is only a small list of foods you truly need to avoid while pregnant, and they fit into two categories: foods that are unsafe and foods that just aren't recommended because they contribute to your toxic load or may affect your baby's development. Again, both lists are short, and while items on the first are absolute no-no's, those on the second may have risks, but the risks may be low. Knowledge is power, and armed with the right information, you can make smart choices about the foods you eat.

I Need My Coffee . . . Please!

First, some good news. You can have coffee while you're pregnant. Yep, I know we're best friends now.

How much coffee is too much? Well, it varies by what study and by what phase the moon is in, apparently, but if you want a normal-sized cup (around eight ounces), go for it. Some studies say you can go up to four cups a day. But even if you *can* have four cups, it doesn't mean you should. Apart from safety concerns, that much caffeine can lead to anxiety, blood sugar fluctuations, and sleep issues. Caffeine can take up to ten hours to clear from your system, so if you consume a cup of coffee at 1:00 p.m., you may still feel the effects until 11:00 p.m. That's more than half of your waking hours spent on the physical and emotional edge. With everything you're going through during pregnancy, do you really need to add fuel to the fire?

Still, we need to feel alive in the morning, so just monitor your intake and take note of how you feel. Like all foods, if possible, buy organic, as conventionally grown coffee beans are high in pesticides and something called mycotoxins, a type of toxin derived from mold.

If it's the caffeine you crave, consider switching to tea. Black and green tea (including matcha) are high in antioxidants and other goodies to sustain and nourish you.

CAFFEINE LEVELS

Caffeine levels can be confusing, and the last thing you need is to be confused when you're battling pregnancy fatigue and don't want to get out of bed. So, here's an at-a-glance table with the approximate caffeine levels of your favorite wake-me-up beverages and snacks. Two hundred milligrams is the recommended daily intake for a pregnant woman, and while I've listed some sugary drinks here for context, I don't advise drinking many of those, because they are full of processed gunk.

DRINK	SIZE (OUNCES)	CAFFEINE LEVEL (MG)
Coffee	8	100
Espresso	2	100
Grande Starbucks latte	16	150
Black tea	8	45
Green tea	8	30 to 50
Chai	8	50
Matcha	12	60 to 70
Dark chocolate	1	20
Decaffeinated coffee	8	2 to 4
Red Bull	8.2	80
Coca-Cola	12	34
Mountain Dew	12	55

Forbidden Foods

This is the short list of the evidence-based no-no's: raw meat, deli meats, rare anything, smoked meats, unpasteurized cheeses, prepackaged salads, and store-bought raw juices. These are the non-negotiables, and here's why. It's not that these foods are "bad" for you; it's that they might be tainted with a pathogen. Since they are undercooked or not cooked at all, the risk of some nasty little bug taking a ride into your gut far outweighs any benefit eating them provides. The specific culprits we're worried about are *E. coli, Toxoplasma gondii, Salmonella,* and *Listeria*, which can cause everything from fatigue, fever, and flu-like symptoms to miscarriage or even death. The Food and Drug

Administration (FDA) has provided such clear guidance on the dangers of foodborne illnesses that I'll leave it to them and the incredibly useful chart on their website, which is listed in the resources section (page 274).

It is often believed that a pregnant woman's immune system is suppressed during early pregnancy (so that her body won't reject a fetus as a "foreign body"), but that is not why some women may feel illnesses come on harder in early pregnancy than in pre-pregnancy. Stanford scientists have discovered that, for the first twelve weeks, the immune response can be *stronger.* That means that if you get sick, your body responds more forcefully, which can lead to you feeling even worse. In your regular life you might just have a twenty-four-hour bout of vomiting, but when you're pregnant, these bad guys can lead to serious complications.

You can't control everything. You may get food poisoning from foods that aren't red flags at all, and it may not be a big deal even if you do. Regardless, if you think you've eaten something that's not agreeing with you (beyond the usual nausea), call your doctor.

Here are other foods you should do your best to avoid, as well as more explanation for why you should steer clear of likely culprits of foodborne illness.

ARTIFICIAL SWEETENERS

These are the first things I recommend my clients omit. Not only do artificial sweeteners disrupt the gut microbiome, but they also increase sugar cravings and appetite (they are two hundred to seven hundred times sweeter than sugar, which makes you need a much higher level of sweetness to feel satisfied). In any amount, saccharin (found in Sweet'N Low) is not safe for expectant moms. It can cross the placenta into fetal tissue, and right now there isn't enough research to determine the risk to your baby. Research is also sparse for sweeteners like aspartame (found in Equal), sucralose (in Splenda), maltitol (in Lesys, among others), acesulfame-K (in Sweet One), and xylitol (found in sugarless gum), which is another reason I recommend cutting them out. Monk fruit has become popular lately because it's derived from a small, green melon, so it is considered a "natural" sugar replacer, but there is no research on whether it's safe in pregnancy. The same goes for stevia, allulose, and erythritol, all of which can also cause GI upset. In general, if small amounts are in, say, your favorite protein powder or electrolyte mix, it's fine, but try to limit them in other contexts.

UNPASTEURIZED CHEESES

You can enjoy all cheeses during pregnancy—*if* they're pasteurized. Bear in mind, however, that the subject of cheese can be confusing. That's because all cheese—even if it's pasteurized—carries some risk of *Listeria,* and pregnant women are seventeen times more likely than the general population to develop an illness (and pass it on to their baby) from *Listeria* exposure. Luckily, the risk of getting listeriosis from cheese is so low—the FDA estimates only one in five million!—that pasteurized cheese is considered safe during pregnancy. In addition, many people believe that all soft cheeses (like Brie, queso fresco, Gorgonzola, and blue) are unpasteurized. This is not true. Many soft cheeses *are* pasteurized, which greatly reduces the chance that you'll get sick from them. If you are confused about whether a cheese is pasteurized, look for the word *pasteurized* before any milk ingredients on the label or ask the local farmer, vendor, or counter salesperson.

RAW, SMOKED, AND DELI MEATS

Like unpasteurized cheese, raw, smoked, and deli meats carry a small risk of listeriosis. Again, it's tiny—only about one thousand six hundred people in the US each year contract illness from *Listeria* (from all sources, not just meat), but I believe it's better to be safe than sorry. Pass on the cold cuts, pâté, meat spreads, and fermented or dry sausages, including chorizo, pepperoni, and salami for now. Refrigeration does not kill *Listeria,* so if you do choose to eat these foods, you can heat them to 165 degrees or higher, which kills pathogens.

PREMADE SALADS AND CUT FRUITS AND VEGETABLES

I love the convenience of a grocery store salad (including chicken, lettuce, and potato salads) and precut, packaged fruits and vegetables—but for the next few months, skip 'em. Because they were assembled in a factory from ingredients that may not have been thoroughly washed, these items have a higher risk of foodborne pathogens, like noroviruses, *Salmonella*, and *E. coli*, than if you prepare them yourself. (Note: if you cook precut vegetables, that will kill any pathogens, so that's a safe alternative.) Produce is the most likely food category to be contaminated with these pathogens, and prepackaged produce causes foodborne illness outbreaks in the US every few years (in contrast, there hasn't been an outbreak from soft cheese since 2017). That salad bar or steam table isn't particularly safe, either. The food may have been out for hours, harboring all kinds of nasties that can get you sick. It's best to avoid them, make your own salads at home, or get one from a restaurant where you know it's been made to order just for you.

Safe and Sometimes Foods

Now, like magic, I'm going to reveal all the foods you thought were off-limits but in fact are available to you—sometimes.

ALCOHOL

You already know that limiting alcohol during pregnancy is recommended. When you drink, alcohol enters your bloodstream, crosses the placenta, and is shared with your fetus. Your baby can process some alcohol, but too much can lead to behavioral and developmental issues, miscarriage, and what's called fetal alcohol spectrum disorder (FASD). The truth is, between the nausea and the exhaustion in the first trimester, you probably won't want it anyway. Regardless, I suggest abstaining entirely for the first few months simply because there is not a lot of research on alcohol use in pregnant women. The few available studies say that one drink a day in the second and third trimesters will have little to no negative effects, and what does matter is what and how quickly you drink. Doing two shots of tequila all at once (please don't do this) is very different from taking a few sips of wine here and there. If you choose to drink at any point, drink slowly, alongside plenty of water and food—especially high-fat foods, which slow the alcohol absorption. But, again, I recommend nothing in the first trimester because the science is not settled. Why take a chance?

FISH

The rules about eating seafood during pregnancy are confusing, not to mention the fact that there are approximately one thousand kinds of fish that you can cook in ten thousand different ways. But my short answer is: Yes! Yes! Yes! Eat fish! Fish is rich in DHA, iodine, zinc, selenium, and B vitamins, meaning that eating it during pregnancy has amazing benefits for both mama and baby. Some fish are high in mercury, but the benefits outweigh the risks. You just need to know what fish to eat and how often.

Aim for two to three times a week. That's roughly twelve ounces a week, which is in line with FDA and Environmental Protection Agency (EPA) guidance.

As for what kind, you can eat many types of fish. Some of my top recommendations are salmon, flaky white fish like cod, sardines, and red snapper. I also like shellfish such as shrimp, scallops, and cooked oysters. As long as your seafood is from a high-quality source there aren't too many restrictions.

The exception here is high-mercury fish, including bigeye tuna, swordfish, shark, marlin, orange roughy, king mackerel, and tilefish. The bigger the fish, the more mercury it absorbs during its lifetime (by eating all the way up and down the food chain, consolidating toxins in its flesh as it goes). Mercury is a neurotoxin that can cause problems in the nervous, digestive, and immune systems. Babies in the womb are especially sensitive, and high levels of mercury exposure lead to long-term neurological effects, including low IQ, decreased test performance, and memory, attention, language, and cognition problems.

A lot of my clients have serious canned tuna cravings and want to know if they can go for it. I experienced those feelings myself. (What I can't say is whether or not I craved tuna *because* it was forbidden. You always want what you can't have!) Here's the deal: most canned tuna, especially high-quality pole or line-caught brands, do not contain any bigeye and instead are made from yellowfin, white, albacore, and skipjack (a tuna-like fish), all considered "medium mercury fish" by the FDA. So the good news is yes, you can have that tuna melt once in a while. Stick to four ounces every few weeks, and look for "pole or line caught," which means that tuna were fished with lines rather than nets, which are notorious for catching—and killing—sharks, dolphins, sea turtles, and other marine life. Pole fishing prevents overfishing and sustains local fishing communities too.

Before we move on, I'm going to put my armor on because I know this will be controversial.

Here we go.

Are you ready?

You can eat sushi.

Yes! It's true. As we discussed earlier, it's not that raw food is the problem, it's that raw food can be a carrier of specific pathogens or bacteria. So there is an inherent risk in eating anything raw, but that risk can be managed if you're comfortable with it. Given that a lot of women can't stand the thought of consuming cooked fish in the first trimester, being able to eat sushi opens up more ways to get those A-plus nutrients in. As always, quality matters, so I only consume raw fish from a well-trusted restaurant or source. No gas station or supermarket sushi, for example.

I do, however, recommend avoiding raw shellfish like oysters and clams. The Centers for Disease Control estimates that eighty thousand illnesses a year are caused by *Vibrio bacteria* that live in warm seawater and frequently infect oysters, so put your raw bar dreams on hold for a few months. However, cooked shellfish (oysters Rockefeller, clams casino, etc.) are a fabulous source of zinc.

I am a lifelong New Yorker, and I love smoked salmon, especially if it's on a hot, toasted bagel with a schmear of cream cheese. I craved it so much during my second pregnancy that I ordered it a few times, forgetting that it was off-limits. (Second-time moms, you can relate.) But there is a risk of *Listeria* poisoning in all smoked fish—unless it's been cooked, like in a casserole—so save the bagel brunch for after you give birth. No lie, I requested a platter of smoked salmon the day I had my son, and I ate every delicious bite.

RUNNY OR SOFT-BOILED EGGS

Eggs are extremely nutritious and a great protein source during pregnancy—and, really, anytime. They also are rich in choline, DHA, and iodine. I'm sure you've heard that while pregnant you should skip the dressing on your Caesar salad because it's made with raw eggs or to fry your eggs into hard bricks. I think that's overkill. Like anything raw or undercooked, runny or raw eggs may contain *Salmonella,* but the chances are low. The Centers for Disease Control (CDC) estimates that only one in every twenty thousand eggs is contaminated with *Salmonella,* and, again, it's not that the egg contains *Salmonella*; it picked it up somewhere on the ride to the grocery store shelves. If you crave a soft-boiled or lightly fried egg, cook it yourself.

SOY

There are a zillion soy products on the market, but they fall into two categories: processed and unprocessed. Processed soy can be found in foods like protein bars, cereals, breads, and veggie burgers, and contain soy protein isolate, while unprocessed soy foods (some of which are fermented) include edamame, miso, natto, tofu, and tempeh. Processed soy contains phytic acid, which makes many vitamins and minerals difficult to absorb, and it may also interfere with estrogen levels.

While soy might seem like a nifty protein alternative for the vegetarians and vegans out there, stick to organic non-GMO tofu and other natural forms of plant-based protein, like legumes/beans, quinoa, nuts, and seeds. Fake meats, like Impossible and Beyond Meat, are made from hyperprocessed soy, so if you are looking for a burger or meat replacement, better options are the kinds made from beans and vegetables.

KOMBUCHA

Kombucha is a probiotic and an antioxidant-rich drink made using tea, sugar, and SCOBY, which stands for "symbiotic cultures of bacteria and yeast." During pregnancy, you want to avoid hard kombucha, which contains a small amount of alcohol produced during the fermenting process. Apart from that, kombucha is unpasteurized, and anything unpasteurized carries a foodborne illness risk, particularly for *Listeria*, although it is rare. There haven't been any *Listeria* outbreaks related to kombucha, but that doesn't mean there aren't isolated cases. Also, kombucha contains caffeine and sugar and is sometimes made with stevia, so check the label carefully to ensure you're not getting too much of something you don't want.

UNPASTEURIZED RAW JUICES

There are few things that are more refreshing and nutrient dense than a raw juice. There's just one issue: drinking them puts you at a higher-than-normal risk for a foodborne illness. The data on outbreaks is difficult to track, but there have been reports of contamination in prepackaged juices. In general, I advise avoiding anything prepackaged, so stick with making your own juice or going to a reputable store or restaurant that presses your drink right in front of you.

A FEW FINAL NOTES ABOUT FOOD SAFETY

Always, always wash your fruits and vegetables, even if the packaging says they've been prewashed. There is a risk (albeit a low one) from store-bought food that could come either from the soil it's grown in or the factory that packaged it. Washing only takes a few moments and can sweep away harmful bacteria, so don't skip it. The FDA offers dozens of other food safety recommendations regarding cleaning, sanitizing, and more, so I highly recommend visiting their website, which they've specially tailored for moms-to-be. I've included a link in the resources section (see page 274).

Finally, this is another plug for organic and local. Most food contamination is the result of the journey that ingredients take to your dinner plate. Local and organic have fewer steps, higher standards, and less opportunity for your tomato to pick up a nasty little passenger.

PANTRY LIST

I give all my pregnant clients this list as soon as they tell me the big news (amazingly, I'm often one of the first people they've told—even before their partners). So, take a picture of this page and hit up the supermarket, farmers market, or wherever you purchase groceries. It might not be the same retail therapy that you're used to, but know you won't regret these purchases.

The list is divided into areas you can easily tackle. You may have much of this on hand already, or you may be starting from scratch. Try to choose organic and grass-fed as budget and access allow, and if you have any allergies or conditions to consider, by all means, steer clear of anything that may exacerbate them. For bread, nuts, fresh fruit, eggs, yogurt, etc., check out your local farms and farmers markets wherever possible.

FREEZER

· Vegetables: Spinach, cauliflower rice, broccoli, string beans, peas, edamame—preferably organic

· Fruit: Unsweetened berries, mango, banana, cherries, pineapple, or whatever fruit you crave—preferably organic

- Veggie burgers: Look for veggie burgers made from whole foods, including vegetables, beans, and grains. Avoid any made with protein isolates (like soy protein isolate) and other ingredients you don't recognize.

- Sliced bread: Sprouted, sourdough, rye, whole-grain, gluten-free (GF), and tortillas

- Bone broth: Look for organic and grass-fed. Bones should be one of the top ingredients, followed by vegetables, herbs, and spices.

SHELF-STABLE

- Oats: Choose quick or old-fashioned (rolled) oats for faster preparation and for baking, or steel-cut for heartier oats (they take longer to cook, but you can make them overnight in a slow cooker). Oats are naturally gluten-free but can be cross-contaminated when grown near wheat, so look for certified gluten-free oats, if preferred.

- Grains: Quinoa, buckwheat, farro, rice

- Beans/lentils (dried or canned): Chickpeas, black beans, white beans (cannellini or great northern), pinto, dried lentils

- Canned fish: Wild salmon, skipjack or light tuna, sardines, crabmeat, anchovies

- High-fiber crackers

- Flour: Almond (GF), oat (GF), whole wheat (pro tip: look for white whole wheat flour; it's made from a lighter type of wheat, so it's whole-grain but closer to white flour in taste and texture)

- Thickeners: Arrowroot flour, cornstarch, tapioca starch

- Pasta: Choose ones made from legumes (GF), quinoa (GF), brown rice (GF), or semolina.

- Organic crushed and diced tomatoes: Look for fire-roasted for extra flavor.

- Tomato sauce

- Tomato paste

- Protein powder: Animal-based ones like whey and beef protein, preferably sweetened with stevia or monk fruit (as opposed to other artificial sweeteners). For plant ones, I recommend hempseed powder.

- Collagen peptides

- Canned coconut milk: Look for a brand made without gums or stabilizers.

- Broth (chicken/vegetable): Organic and low-sodium

- Dried dates

- Cacao nibs

- Cacao powder

- Brewer's yeast: Look for debittered.

- Baking soda

- Baking powder: Look for a brand that doesn't include aluminum. If you're avoiding gluten, check the label, because some are made with wheat starch. You want "double-acting" baking powder, which means that it reacts when it hits liquid and again when it hits heat.

FATS AND OILS

- Extra-virgin olive oil

- Avocado oil and spray

- Coconut oil: Look for unrefined or virgin coconut oil. If you don't like the taste of coconut, pick a more neutral oil, like avocado, instead.

- Toasted sesame oil: This is a finishing oil, which means you drizzle it on at the end. Do not cook with it.

- Pesto

- Ghee: This is butter that's been clarified to remove the milk solids.

- Unsalted butter: Preferably grass-fed and/or organic

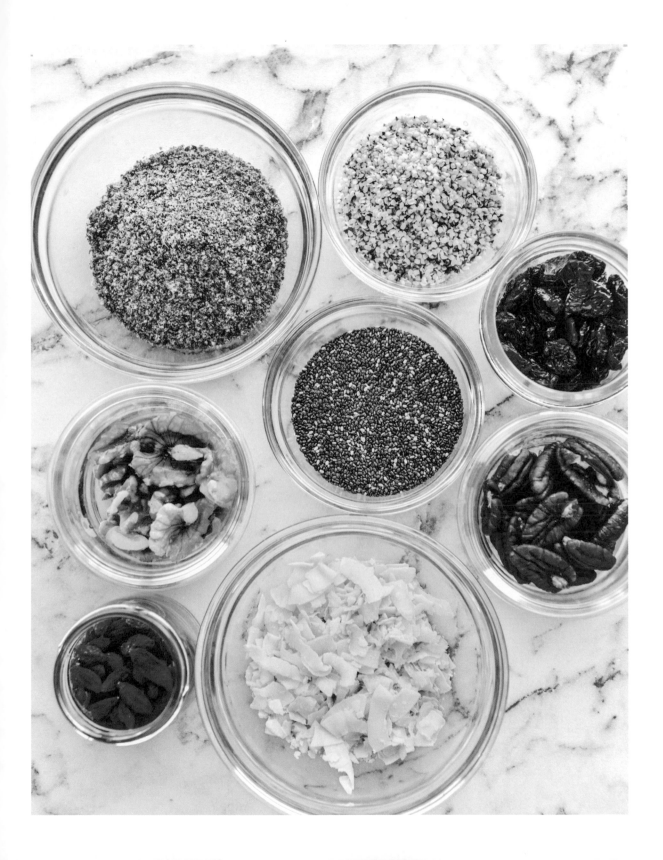

- Nut/seed butters: These include peanut, almond, cashew, and coconut butters, and tahini. The ingredient list on the label should just be nuts/seeds or nuts/seeds plus salt.

SEEDS AND NUTS

- Pumpkin seeds

- Sesame seeds

- Sunflower seeds

- Hempseed hearts

- Ground flaxseed

- Chia seeds

- Dry roasted walnuts, almonds, cashews, macadamia nuts, pecans, pistachios

- Unsweetened flaked coconut

VINEGAR/CONDIMENTS

- Coconut aminos (gluten-/soy-free), tamari (GF soy sauce), or soy sauce (low-sodium)

- Miso: This fermented soybean paste will keep for a long time in the fridge. The lighter in color, the milder and less salty.

- Apple cider vinegar

- Rice vinegar: Look for unseasoned (seasoned usually has added sugar).

- Balsamic vinegar

- Red wine vinegar

- Mayonnaise: Look for a brand made with avocado oil.

- Mustard: Dijon, yellow

- Hot sauces: Sriracha, buffalo sauce, or whatever variety you like

- Barbecue sauce: Look for brands sweetened with fruit or small amounts of natural sweeteners like honey or maple syrup.

- Canned chipotles in adobo

REFRIGERATOR/PERISHABLES

- Eggs: Large, preferably pasture-raised and/or organic. Eggshell color doesn't matter.

- Yogurt: Full fat, plain

- Cottage cheese: Full fat, plain

- Avocados

- Vegetables galore! Whatever is in season and you like. Think greens (kale, spinach, mixed greens, arugula), cruciferous veggies (broccoli, Brussels sprouts, cauliflower), zucchini, asparagus, string beans, mushrooms, cabbage (green and purple), snap peas, snow peas, root veggies (carrots, beets, parsnips, sweet potatoes, turnips), bell peppers, cucumbers, fennel, tomatoes, celery, winter squash (butternut, acorn, delicata, spaghetti).

- Fresh herbs: Parsley, dill, cilantro, basil

- Fermented vegetables: Sauerkraut, pickles (buy refrigerated ones, which should say "raw" and/or "fermented" on the label, to make sure you get the gut health benefits)

- Fruit: Whatever you like that's in season—bananas, kiwi, berries (blueberries, raspberries, strawberries, blackberries), apples, pears, citrus (lemons, limes, grapefruit, oranges, tangerines), melons, pineapples, mangoes, peaches, plums, nectarines, cherries

- Pasteurized cheese: Parmigiano-Reggiano, feta, goat, cheddar, mozzarella, Gouda, Muenster

- Tortillas: Corn or flour

- Tofu: Organic, non-GMO, extra firm

- Fresh ginger: Keep it in the freezer; mince or grate it frozen, no need to defrost first.

- Olives/capers

- Full-fat dairy and/or nondairy varieties like almond, cashew, macadamia, and oat milk: Look for minimal ingredients without gums or fillers.

- Shallots, onions, red onions, garlic

SWEETENERS

- Raw honey

- Maple syrup

- Coconut sugar

- Date sugar

- Molasses

SEASONINGS

- Fine sea salt, flaky sea salt, kosher salt

- Ground cinnamon (preferably Ceylon)

- Ground cumin

- Ground coriander

- Garlic powder

- Onion powder

- Ground ginger

- Chili powder

- Paprika: Sweet, hot, smoked

- Dried oregano

- Ground nutmeg

- Dried thyme

- Dried bay leaf

- Turmeric

- Seasoning blends: Choose the ones you like—taco seasoning, Italian seasoning, curry powder, za'atar, pumpkin pie spice, Cajun seasoning.

- Ground black pepper (or peppercorns, if you have a grinder)

- Extracts: Pure vanilla, lemon, almond

CHAPTER 4

NOURISHING AND PROTECTING BABY

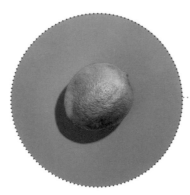

YOUR BABY IS THE SIZE OF A LIME AROUND WEEK TWELVE.

Now that we've covered *you*, it's time to move on to the little one who's growing by the day. Let's start with some good news. The food that nourishes you will go a long way toward nourishing your baby. Your nutritional intake is a baseline for their development and ensures they thrive, both in the womb and once they are born.

That being said, even if you already eat a generally healthy diet, there are a bunch of foods you'll want to add—and others to be wary of. This second part is important. Chronic allergic illnesses in children are everywhere—and on the rise. For example, the CDC reports that 5.8 percent of children in the United States have food allergies, while 10.8 percent have eczema. The American Lung Association states that a whopping one out of eight children suffers from asthma. While there are often a variety of causes, these conditions are connected to the developing immune system, which is linked to the microbiome. Because the microbiome is so inextricable from the diet, there are steps you can take in your pregnancy to reduce the likelihood of some of these issues.

My son had eczema and food allergies and still has "sensitive" lungs, so this subject is personal. I have worked hard to understand the why of these conditions in kids, and I've been fortunate to learn from some amazing practitioners over the years. Thankfully, my son has come a long way. He no longer has egg and tree nut allergies, can tolerate certain peanut products, rarely has an itch or eczema flare-up, and doesn't need an inhaler when he has a cold. But if I had known during my pregnancy what I know now, I would have made some different decisions.

Let's dive in.

NUTRIENTS FOR YOUR LITTLE ONE

Even when the fetus is just a few cells, it still needs nutrients. Think of it like this—that little seed is basically a cell-dividing and cell-producing machine working in overdrive, and it requires fuel. Pretty cool, right? So what are the key nutrients and foods to help that tiny machine divide and conquer? In chapter 2, we talked about these vitamins and minerals in the context of prenatals and food sources. In chapter 3, we discussed the macronutrients you should consume—proteins, fats, and carbs—and the particular nutrients contained in each. I encourage you to revisit those chapters and charts to understand their benefits to you and your growing baby. Remember: what's good for mom is good for the little person inside her.

PREGNANCY AND YOUR BABY'S MICROBIOME

The early months are crucial for the development of your baby's microbiome, which is the tiny world of bacteria, viruses, and other microbes that aid in digestion, metabolism, immunity, mood, brain health, thyroid function, and

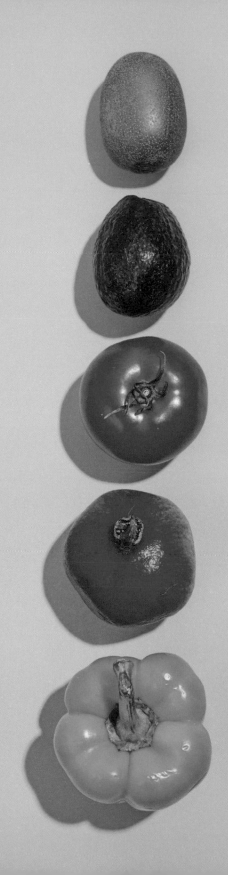

growth. There are nearly one hundred trillion gut microorganisms in your body that, collectively, weigh 4.4 pounds. That's about equal to the weight of a standard-sized brick. Those sky-high numbers of colony forming units (CFUs) in probiotic drinks (five billion!) make a bit more sense now, right?

During pregnancy and childbirth, a mother passes her microbiome directly to her baby through the placenta and umbilical cord, the mouth (oral bacteria that go into the bloodstream), and the birth canal, and breastmilk and skin-to-skin contact after birth. If something's coming through the umbilical cord, it's probably because you ate it or were otherwise exposed to it in your environment. Whatever you consume has an impact on your fetus's gut, and a healthy microbiome decreases the chances of immune-related diseases like food allergies, eczema, and IBS.

How do you create a healthy microbiome for yourself, which will then help your little one? First and foremost, by eating a well-balanced diet. This includes the following:

· Avoiding excess sugar, preservatives, chemicals (like pesticides), and artificial sweeteners. Too much of these things can cause dysbiosis (an imbalance), which is the overgrowth of harmful microbes or depletion of healthy microbes.

· Fiber! Eating a variety of fresh, colorful, nutrient-dense fruits and vegetables and healthy legumes and whole grains promotes a healthy, diverse microbiome.

· Eating probiotic-rich fermented foods like miso, sauerkraut, kimchi, pickled veggies (look for the words *raw* or *unpasteurized* on the label and ensure they're not heat-treated, like your average hamburger or sandwich pickles), kefir, and yogurt. (But stay away from high-alcohol-content kombucha.)

· Eating prebiotic-rich foods, which stimulate the growth of healthy bacteria. Prebiotic foods include artichokes, bananas, asparagus, apples, onions, and garlic (avoid garlic if it gives you acid reflux).

· Taking a probiotic supplement, especially in the third trimester. In fact, you may want to consider an infant probiotic once the little one arrives (talk to your doctor, of course). This is especially true if you need to take antibiotics for any reason during pregnancy, as they will wipe out much of your microbiome.

TOXINS AND PREGNANCY

While we always kept a fairly "natural" house, when I became pregnant with Julian, I became hypervigilant and got rid of almost everything that was not organic or "clean," for lack of a better word. This included all our cleaning supplies, toothpaste, makeup, and hair products.

My husband was just as deep in the rabbit hole—maybe more so—and soon it became overwhelming to remain constantly vigilant. But I also knew that we are exposed in ways our parents never were, whether that's mile-long food labels filled with chemicals we can't pronounce or microplastics that are pervasive in our drinking water. However, we all need to strike a balance between being paranoid and living our lives. Even small changes add up and can make a difference.

Still, my pendulum swung a bit too far in the paranoid direction, and today I know that most of these issues should not keep you up at night. As you read this section and feel any anxiety setting in, remember:

1. You can find something "wrong" with every single food item, including kale and water. Studies have even found trace amounts of lead and cadmium in cacao and dark chocolate. Remember that perfect is by far the greatest enemy of good. No one living in our society can prevent 100 percent of negative environmental exposures during pregnancy. Do what you can, what you can afford, and what's right for you. Don't put pressure on yourself to take on more than you can handle, because I know you're making a million other educated, loving choices for your baby. Maybe you want to clear out everything at once or just dip a toe in the water and make some small (but still impactful) changes. Today, I do my best for my kids, but I do not let these types of concerns consume me. That said, if you're looking for more specific guidance on items you know may carry small risks, simply don't eat them every day to avoid the possibility of building up a toxin's concentration in your body. Can pregnant women still eat dark chocolate? Absolutely! Should they eat it in unlimited amounts? Probably not. Keep these scientific headlines (there are a lot of them, often contradictory) in perspective.

2. Nothing is mandatory. I am simply providing information. Take from it what you want.

3. Science is evolving. Some of what I write is fact, some of it is based on my experience, and some of it is debatable or hypothetical.

To help you sort through what chemicals you should look out for—and why they matter—I've created another chart, which follows on page 94. Bear in mind that the subject of environmental toxins is so far-reaching that I encourage you to dive into the resources I've listed (see page 274) if you want to go deeper. You could write a book on these alone—and many have.

The items listed in this chart are called endocrine-disrupting chemicals (EDCs). There are over eight hundred EDCs, and they are found in herbicides, pesticides, plastics, detergents, toys, some metals, stain repellants, nonstick pans, flame retardants, and cosmetics. EDCs interfere with your body's endocrine function, which is the network of glands that secrete hormones that regulate reproduction, energy levels, mood, sleep function, and metabolism. These glands are in full force during pregnancy, so best not to mess with them.

CHEMICAL	WHAT IT IS	WHERE IT'S FOUND
Bisphenol A (BPA)	A chemical used in the production of polycarbonate plastics	Water bottles, baby bottles, food cans, bottle tops, plastic food containers
Fluoride	An odorless, tasteless chemical compound often added to toothpaste or drinking water to strengthen and protect teeth	Toothpaste, tap water
Aluminum	A soft, bendable chemical element that, in excess amounts, cannot be excreted by the body and lodges in the bones, brain, spleen, muscles, and other organs	Aluminum foil, deodorant, aluminum cans, antacids
Pesticides	Chemicals used to attack the nervous systems of insects and cause them to die	Gardening sprays, bug sprays, and large-scale sprays and additives used in agricultural areas
Phthalates	Also called plasticizers, they make plastics more durable.	Packaging, tubing, vinyl flooring, personal care products, detergents
Flame retardants	In scientific terms, they're polybrominated diphenyl ethers (PBDEs), and they attach to household dust and disrupt thyroid function	Furniture, carpeting, even pajamas

Take a deep breath. I'm going to discuss how to easily avoid or minimize these chemicals during pregnancy, or—as I like to say—control the controllables. At home, I try to make swaps when possible but don't obsess when I am out of my house. I make small changes here and there but don't go on a search-and-destroy mission against every possibly toxic product in my life once a month.

You can adopt a few of these suggestions or none at all. My goal is to simplify the overwhelming into some actionable items. Take it one step at a time.

Plastics

· Use glass, silicone, or stainless-steel food containers instead of plastic containers. Especially avoid heating your food in plastic. If you order takeout, plate it, then heat it.

· Swap plastic water bottles for stainless steel or glass.

Cosmetics

· According to the EWG, one out of twenty-four women is exposed to personal-care products that can have adverse effects on the reproductive system and babies in the womb. Avoid products with "fragrance" on the ingredient list, and consult the EWG database for a long list of nontoxic cosmetics and hygiene products.

Water

· If you have a well or a cistern, you should have your water tested by a certified lab and install a water filter designed for well water, whether under the counter or for the whole home. If you use municipal water, I also recommend filtering the water. There are some very low-cost, easy-to-install, under-the-sink filters in lieu of using a pitcher filter. The EWG has a great guide.

Foods

· Try to choose organic when possible (for more on this, see page 58) to reduce pesticides.

· When making popcorn, swap microwavable popcorn for stove top, which is easy and fun to make. The bags used in microwave popcorn contain EDCs.

- Avoid or eat fewer mercury-rich foods (see page 76).

- If you drink tea, swap plastic tea bags for loose-leaf tea or tea bags that don't contain EDCs.

Cooking and Cleaning

- Replace nonstick pans (this was a tough one for me) with stainless steel or cast iron pans. Change out any aluminum utensils, baking sheets, or roasting pans for stainless steel, cast iron, or silicone.

- When cooking, use your kitchen range hood to help keep the air as clean as possible. If you don't have a hood, open a window and turn on a fan.

- Use unbleached parchment paper or silicone instead of aluminum foil when baking or roasting.

- Upgrade your cleaning supplies to environmentally safe products that don't contain chemicals or fragrances like formaldehyde and boric acid. Consult the resources section (see page 274) for a comprehensive list from the EWG, and keep in mind that words like "green," "natural," and "organic" don't mean anything when it comes to labels on cleaning supplies. You should always look at the actual ingredients.

- Invest in air filters that will remove toxins from the air and eliminate dust and germs that might make you sick. Don't get too in the weeds with research; just make sure it has a HEPA filter.

Health and Hygiene

- Switch to an aluminum-free deodorant. Yes, this was a tough one for me too.

- I know you're not two years old, but don't swallow toothpaste. Consider switching to a fluoride-free variety during pregnancy. Little secret . . . it's the brushing that cleans your teeth, not just the paste, so natural ones work just as well as the extra-minty stuff.

- Use sunscreen that contains zinc oxide or titanium dioxide rather than chemical ingredients like oxybenzone or retinyl palmitate.

Garden and Yard

· Avoid using chemical-based pesticides in your yard or garden. This is especially important during the first trimester, when your baby's nervous system is developing.

I'll say it again: do your best, and do not beat yourself up over the things you have around your house or have put into your body. You're going to microwave something in a plastic container, you're going to be thirsty and forget your reusable bottle, and you're going to breathe air that's polluted, because that's our world. Just remember that every small choice and positive change makes a difference. The best results often come from gradual, sustainable shifts rather than one big, dramatic move.

SECTION TWO: THE SECOND TRIMESTER

You made it . . . out of the first trimester. Welcome back to the world. First, well done, and if it was a cinch, then well done too. For a lot of you, the second trimester will be a golden period: you made it through a really difficult adjustment—both physically and emotionally—and now you have the lay of the land. Don't get me wrong, you may not feel like life is all sunshine and rainbows, but chances are you've experienced a substantial shift. Foods you couldn't bear to look at are appealing again, and the thought of cooking or going to a restaurant doesn't send you under the covers. You're able to keep your eyes open for more than a few hours a day, and, hopefully, you're worrying less that any little thing could harm your baby. Yay for progress! You'll soon notice a more defined bump and some weight gain, and you'll get to soak up all the fun and excitement of telling people that, yes, you're pregnant!

The second trimester is the time to focus on *you* and *your needs*, so we'll cover how to welcome food back into your life (hooray!), create structure around meals and snacks, and control your blood sugar and cravings. I'll also discuss some of the yucky symptoms that may still pop up and the tests that will help you avoid or manage serious conditions—but for the most part, the second trimester can be fun. I'll try to make the nutritional side of things more enjoyable too.

CHAPTER 5

MEALS, SNACKS, AND
SATISFYING MAMA

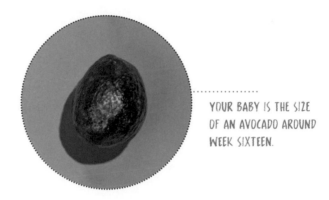

YOUR BABY IS THE SIZE
OF AN AVOCADO AROUND
WEEK SIXTEEN.

The second trimester is an incredible time of change and surprises for you and the little person inside you. Your baby grows from about the size of a lime at week twelve to an avocado at week sixteen, and by the end of the second trimester, they'll be as long as an ear of corn. The delicate fluttering of butterfly wings inside you will transform into full-on karate-style kicks, and some of you will notice sharp elbows, dance parties (every time my husband came home), flips and turns, and adorable hiccups. Your baby will grow working ears, visible hair, fingerprints, and footprints, and will even begin to suck their thumb. Their lungs develop, their eyes move, and they pack fat onto their developing muscles and hardening bones.

You're changing too. When your appetite comes back, it also makes a pretty cool pivot: food satisfies you in ways that it didn't in the first trimester *and* even before you were pregnant. You may want to eat at different times, you'll definitely want to eat more, and you may find yourself trying to satisfy some wild cravings. In this chapter, we'll dive into how you can tailor your meals to suit your needs and desires. This is the golden trimester, so your food should be perfectly suited for *you*.

NOURISHMENT FOR MAMA AND BABY

Let's start with the satisfying part: food. In the second trimester, food is like a long-lost friend who just moved in next door. You're going to be spending a lot of time catching up, and that's a good thing, because right now mama and baby need tons of nourishment from nutrient-dense foods. As we dive into how to eat, what to eat, and why, I cannot stress enough that you are going to eat a lot—or at least more than you're used to. Hunger will just be *different*. It can be jarring, especially if you barely wanted to touch food for the last three months, but you get used to it (*I'm hungry again!?*). A little bit of thought and planning goes a long way. So let's jump in.

SETTING EXPECTATIONS

The main questions I get are "How much should I eat?" and "When?" Like with everything in pregnancy and life, there is no one-size-fits-all answer. You have to listen to your body. While at first that might have felt impossible, by now you're probably noticing patterns, consistencies, and other tells to guide you. More often than not, your cravings reveal the nutrients your body and baby need.

Pre-pregnancy, maybe you were a three-meals-a-day and no-snacks type, or maybe you ate multiple small meals. However you used to roll, there are some basic frameworks I believe you should now try to follow. The first thing to know is that you should throw your old expectations about mealtimes and snacks out the window. Pregnancy is like a trip to the moon and back.

BREAKFAST OF CHAMPIONS

Let's start at the very beginning. **Eat breakfast, and do it right.** While your body was resting overnight, your baby was still growing and devouring the calories and nutrients you took in during the days, weeks, and months before. Refueling first thing is vital to set the tone for the rest of the day. From a nutrient perspective, eating a healthy breakfast also stabilizes your blood sugar levels, combats GI issues like acid reflux, and prevents you from feeling on edge. In your old life, maybe you were a breakfast skipper; I cannot stress enough that those days are gone.

What does a substantial, healthy breakfast look like? During pregnancy, protein is a must at every meal, but it should be center stage at breakfast. Why? After we fast all night, our bodies are ultrasensitive to glucose, and that means that what you eat first will get digested super fast. As such, you need protein to prevent the blood sugar spike that you'd get from, say, a carb-heavy bowl of cereal. A protein at breakfast will also help regulate your blood sugar throughout the day, preventing those spikes and plummets even later on. If you have a sugary, carb-heavy breakfast that lacks protein, or no breakfast, you're in for a massive crash by lunch. Before the little one, you might have been able to manage, but now these peaks and valleys are amplified.

With protein as the base, you'll add some fat (avocado, nuts, nut butter) or cook with butter, olive oil, coconut oil, or avocado oil. Give yourself extra points for fiber (veggies, chia seeds, ground flaxseed) and, as an option, some form of starch (toast, oats, grains, potatoes) or fruit (fresh or frozen).

When it comes to portions, as always, trust your body. If you feel full, you most likely are, and if you are still hungry, well, that's your body telling you something. Listen to its cues, especially in the beginning of the second trimester as you're getting your food legs back. Soon, knowing your body's new rhythms will be second nature.

HERE ARE TWENTY-ONE EASY BREAKFAST IDEAS THAT ARE DESIGNED WITH A SECOND TRIMESTER MAMA IN MIND.

1. **Greek yogurt bowl:** Full-fat, plain Greek yogurt (or unsweetened coconut yogurt if you're dairy-free) with seeds of choice (hemp, ground flax, pumpkin, sesame), one teaspoon of honey, and mixed berries

2. **Baked oatmeal (see page 266):** Topped with plain full-fat Greek yogurt, tahini, or nut butter

3. **Toast plus:** Sourdough toast topped with avocado, a sprinkle of hempseed hearts, and eggs of any style

4. **Veggie frittata (see page 193):** One slice, using any combo of veggies and adding cheese or herbs, if desired; served with optional whole wheat, sprouted, or sourdough toast with mashed avocado

5. **Green smoothie (see page 191)**

6. **Blueberry tahini smoothie (see page 192)**

7. **Tropical smoothie (see page 192)**

8. **Green waffles (see page 197):** Topped with honey-butter compote or nut butter, plus a little jam, like the chia jam included on page 198

9. **Breakfast broth:** Bone Broth (page 247) with poached or soft-boiled eggs, zucchini noodles (softened in the broth), topped with Parmesan

10. **Chia seed pudding:** One fourth of a cup of chia seeds mixed with one and a fourth cups of milk of choice or canned coconut milk, one teaspoon of vanilla extract, two teaspoons of maple syrup, shaken and left for 15 minutes in the refrigerator, then shaken again and left in the refrigerator for at least an hour or overnight; topped with fruit of choice or nuts of choice (serves two)

11. **Overnight oats:** Half a cup of dry rolled oats combined with half a cup milk of choice, one fourth of a cup of plain full-fat Greek yogurt, one tablespoon of chia seeds, one teaspoon of maple syrup, and a pinch of fine sea salt; left overnight in the refrigerator; topped in the morning with shredded, unsweetened coconut flakes, nut butter or nuts, and fruit of choice

12. **Veggie omelet:** One cup of veggies of choice (mushrooms, bell peppers, spinach, kale, and onions are all great) sautéed in olive oil until soft; cooked with two whisked eggs until set; served with avocado, toast, or fruit of choice

13. **Fruity cottage cheese:** Full-fat cottage cheese with cut-up fruit of choice (berries, kiwi, apples, etc.), one tablespoon of chia seeds, and slivered almonds

14. **Savory cottage cheese:** Full-fat cottage cheese with sliced Persian cucumbers and grape/cherry tomatoes, topped with nut of choice and seasoned with fine sea salt, pepper, everything bagel seasoning, or fresh chives

15. **Veggie egg bowl:** Roasted broccoli or sautéed spinach, tomatoes, and chickpeas topped with eggs and cheese of choice, like feta or goat

16. **Eggs any style:** Add sautéed spinach, avocado, and a piece of toast

17. **Lentils topped with egg(s):** Add avocado or greens

18. **Breakfast burrito:** One wrap stuffed with mashed avocado, scrambled eggs, refried beans, and salsa

19. **PB&J:** Toast topped with nut butter of choice, berry chia jam (see page 198), and a sprinkle of hempseed hearts

20. **Carrot cake muffins (see page 206):** Topped with nut butter or paired with an egg or two

21. **Two-ingredient banana/egg pancakes:** One mashed ripe banana combined with two eggs, plus a little vanilla extract and cinnamon, to make the batter; cooked like pancakes in butter, avocado oil, or coconut oil

ANATOMY OF A SMOOTHIE

One of my favorite ways to build a satisfying breakfast that packs in a lot of nutrients is to make a smoothie. Smoothies provide fiber and much-needed fruits, vegetables, and proteins and they hydrate you. They're a delicious way to shake up a meal (pun intended).

But not all smoothies are created equal from a nutritional perspective, and some can spike your blood sugar if they're not nutritionally complete. Before you plug in your blender, remember to think of a smoothie as a meal in a glass and build it the same way. It should include a protein, fat, and fiber. Here are some of the best options for each:

PROTEIN

- Nuts/nut butter
- Seeds
- Yogurt/kefir
- Cow's or goat's milk
- Hempseed hearts (three tablespoons = ten grams of protein)
- Collagen
- Protein powder

FRUIT (INCLUDE ANYWHERE FROM HALF A CUP TO TWO CUPS)

- Banana
- Berries
- Kiwi
- Cherries
- Mango
- Pineapple
- Apple
- Pear
- Melon
- Dragon fruit
- Acai

FAT (ONE TO TWO TABLESPOONS)

- Coconut: shredded, unsweetened, or in oil form
- Avocado (half an avocado)
- Nuts/nut butter or seeds/seed butter

FIBER (ONE TO TWO TABLESPOONS)

- Chia seeds
- Flaxseed, ground
- Wheat germ
- Psyllium husk

VEGGIES (ONE TO TWO HANDFULS)

- Spinach
- Kale
- Chard
- Cauliflower
- Cucumber
- Carrots
- Beets

LIQUID BASE (THREE-FOURTHS TO ONE CUP)

- Milk of choice (cow, goat, almond, macadamia, coconut, oat)
- Coconut water
- Water

OPTIONAL ADD-INS

- Cinnamon
- Ginger
- Cacao powder
- Cacao nibs
- Goji berries
- Mint
- Basil

BUILDING A BETTER SNACK

Snack anxiety is a thing. Are you snacking too much? Too little? Too early? Too late? During pregnancy, and especially in the second trimester, snacking—when done wisely—is your friend. It's going to get you through the day, creating a supportive bridge between meals.

But how does one snack "wisely" when you're hungry and fatigued, and your options are the random abandoned items in your office pantry, whatever's closest to the convenience store checkout, or the leftovers from your preschooler's lunch box? And how can you get over the feeling that snacking is unhealthy, gluttonous, or bad?

I like to think of snacks as mini meals because they are. It's time to shift your mindset and know that snacks are just as essential as full meals, as long as they're nutritious and filling. You'll find a full list of DIY snacks on page 115, but let's make things easy to start. Here's the formula:

P (protein) + F (fiber) + F (fat) − S (stress) = Satisfied Mama

A snack should consist of a minimum of two out of these three: protein, fiber, and fat. And remember, one thing that is completely forbidden from any snack is stress.

- **Protein:** Hard-boiled eggs, nuts, nut butter, seeds (pumpkin, hemp), beans (including hummus or bean dip), chickpeas, and an animal protein like turkey jerky or a dairy source like full-fat yogurt, cottage cheese, or cheese

- **Fiber:** Fruits, vegetables, high-fiber crackers, legumes (chickpeas, beans, lentils), and seeds like chia and ground flax

- **Fat:** Dairy (full-fat yogurt, cottage cheese, cheese), avocados, nuts and nut butter, seeds (pumpkin, hemp), coconut, and oils (olive, coconut, avocado)

Put them together and you're looking at veggies with hummus, cheese and crackers, apples with cashew butter, trail mix made with pistachios, macadamia nuts, and dried fruit, or avocado toast. As long as the formula stays intact, you can mix and match it to suit your tastes.

Now that we've covered the formulation, let's discuss the frequency. If you consider a snack a mini meal, aim to plate it, sit down, and enjoy it. I know what it's like coming home ravenous, opening up the cabinets, and going to town. No guilt; I've been there. But eating mindfully will keep you from turning a healthy snack intended to energize you into something that slows you down. With that in mind, timing depends on your habits and schedule. Do you wake up at 5:00 a.m. so you can be at work by 6:30 a.m.? You're probably going to need a morning snack. Are you a night owl? Consider snacking at night.

Here's a sample snack schedule:

- **Morning snack:** Morning snacks work best for those who eat breakfast early and are genuinely hungry a few hours later. The goal is to take the edge off, not to fill up so much that you skip lunch. Consider both a bigger breakfast and, if you're still hungry, a snack.

- **Afternoon snack:** This is the day's most substantial snack. The gap between lunch and dinner is typically wide (meaning five-plus hours), so you'll likely need a pick-me-up. You may find one small snack satisfies you, or you may have a second lunch at three or four, like I did. Your snack strategy might also include two smaller snacks at, say, three and five thirty.

- **After dinner:** Here's where good eating hygiene comes into play, because nighttime puts a lot of us into a habit-forming emotional eating zone. If you tend toward emotional eating, think about why you're reaching into the fridge by using what's called the HALT strategy: ask yourself, Am I Hungry, Anxious (or Angry), Lonely, or Tired? Unless it's a genuine H, you're in emotional eating territory, and taking a beat to identify the non-H cause can help you put down the popcorn before you've cleaned out the bowl.

In addition, be mindful of food products that are tough to portion (like bags of chips, popcorn, cereal, or salty nuts). If you are craving them, that's cool; just aim to plate your snack (or separate it into smaller containers) and include

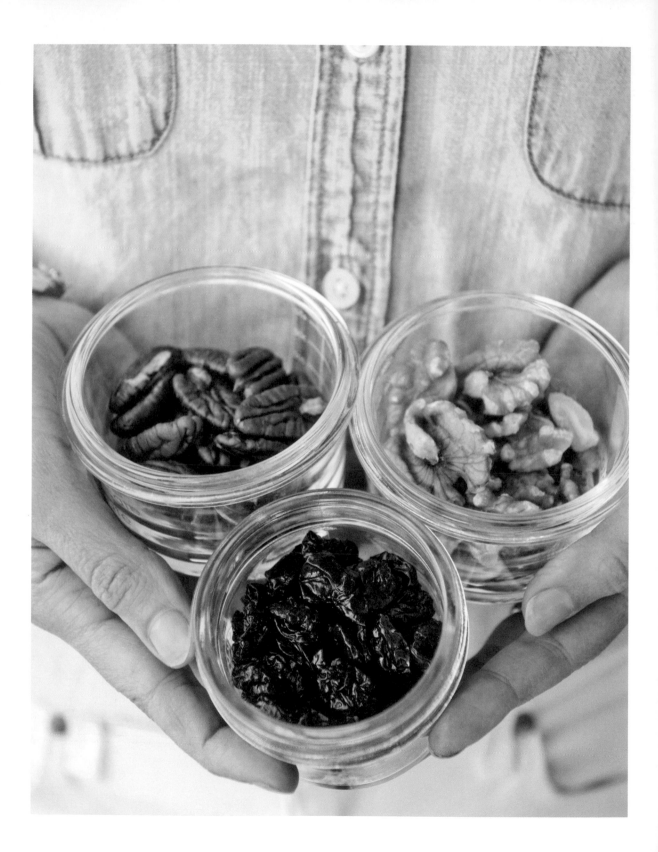

protein. The goal here is to find the foods that are satisfying and that you can portion control. I've included some great snack and mini meal ideas at the end of this section (see page 115).

LUNCH

Lunch is hard, especially if you are at work or are short on time, so here are my strategies to keep lunch interesting—and simple.

- **Practice partial meal prep:** You don't need to spend all day Sunday prepping. Instead, take an hour or so on the weekend to ready a few foods that can easily be assembled into complete meals. This may include chopping vegetables, boiling eggs, or making a big pot of quinoa or lentil veggie soup.

- **Rely on quick and easy proteins:** Some you will need to cook in advance (like eggs, egg salad, meatballs, ground meats, lentils, and rotisserie chicken—which you can shred and store for even quicker meals); others are shelf stable, like beans, chickpeas (if you buy canned beans, drain and rinse them ahead of time, then keep them in the fridge for three to four days), roasted chickpea snacks, and canned salmon and sardines; and others you can pop in the freezer, like organic chicken nuggets. Pick a few of these easy protein options to put into the rotation each week.

- **Rely on roasted vegetables:** I recommend batch cooking vegetables such as broccoli, cauliflower, Brussels sprouts, asparagus, carrots, and zucchini and keeping them in a glass container so all you need to do is heat and enjoy. You can also keep raw and/or fermented veggies (cucumbers, carrots, peppers, snap peas, etc.) on hand for salads or simple sides. Any way you cut it, you should aim to cover half your plate with vegetables.

- **Add carbohydrates:** Batch cook grains, like rice or farro, and/or roasted potatoes (any color) to have on hand for easy grain bowls.

- **Utilize leftovers:** When you're cooking dinner, double the servings so you'll have leftovers for the next day. That's how I roll.

EASY LUNCH IDEAS

The recipe section includes more easy-to-prepare lunch recipes, but here are some of my basic go-tos for the midday meal.

- **Avocado/egg salad:** Combine avocado, hard-boiled eggs, diced cucumber, chopped onion, and salt/pepper/spices of choice. Serve on top of greens, high-fiber crackers, or toast or in a wrap.

- **Mashed chickpea salad:** Combine mashed chickpeas with hummus or avocado. You can serve this on top of greens, high-fiber crackers, or toast or in a wrap.

- **Open-faced cottage cheese or ricotta cheese toast:** Top with cucumbers and cherry tomatoes

- **Avocado toast with egg(s):** Avocado mashed on toast plus egg(s) any way you want, seasoned with salt/pepper/red pepper flakes

- **Salmon salad**: One can of salmon with mayo over high-fiber crackers, greens, or toast

- **Stuffed sweet potato:** Use black beans, cheese, and broccoli

- **Lettuce wrap:** Wrap ground meat (turkey/chicken/beef), pickles, veggies, and hummus or avocado

- **Veggie burger:** Add hummus with a side of veggies/salad

- **Soup:** Think chicken veggie, butternut squash, chili, lentil, or minestrone, paired with a slice of toast topped with cheese, avocado, or hummus

- **Grain bowls:** Throw together a precooked grain of choice and a protein (hard-boiled eggs, shredded chicken, chickpeas, or beans), veggies, and fat of choice (avocado, tahini, or pesto)

- **Veggie omelet or make-ahead frittata (see page 193):** Add greens of choice

- **Cheese, spinach, and chicken quesadilla:** Use whole wheat or grain-free wraps

- **Meatballs (see page 251):** Sauce them with marinara or pesto and put them on spaghetti squash, pasta, or zucchini noodles or throw them on a salad or pair them with sautéed spinach

DINNER

It's like lunch, but later! Your same meal goals apply here: half your plate veggies, a fourth protein, a fat, and an optional starch.

Here's the embarrassing truth: I meal plan all day for my clients—I'm *really* good at it—but by the time my own family's dinner rolls around . . . not so much. What I've found works best to get food on the table is what I call the weeknight shuffle. Instead of planning each meal each week, I create theme nights. Sticking to these themes—with the flexibility to try new recipes—makes it fun for the whole family and makes your life (and mental load) about ten times easier.

For example:

- Monday: Fish

- Tuesday: Tacos

- Wednesday: Sheet pan chicken

- Thursday: Slow cooker

- Friday: Grain bowl

- Saturday: Eat out/order in

- Sunday: Pasta

DESSERTS

There are so few true indulgences in life; we should cherish them. My philosophy on dessert is pretty straightforward: always go for the real thing (skip the fakes full of artificial ingredients and bad-for-you sweeteners), and then enjoy it in a positive, mindful way. There is a difference between downing a pint of ice cream on your couch and going to an ice cream store with a friend to catch up over a cone. Aim to eat sweets after a meal that contains protein, fat, and fiber, which will reduce the sugar spike. Eat a reasonable amount until you feel full and satisfied. Most critically, don't feel guilty about treating yourself in a loving way. Dessert can be both an indulgence and an act of self-care.

A special word about chocolate. Chocolate is my favorite food (it comprises its own food group as far as I'm concerned). If you also have a chocolate tooth, aim for dark varieties (anything above 72 percent, but I encourage you to try 80 or even 90 percent). Keep your intake to one to two squares a day, and bear in mind that chocolate contains caffeine, so pay attention to how you feel after; if you're having trouble sleeping or getting a buzz, you may need to have this particular treat earlier in the day. (As I mentioned on page 92, chocolate also contains trace amounts of some metals, though this is a small risk.) If you have bad acid reflux, chocolate will also make you feel worse. I'm so sorry! There are so many other sweet treats you can and should enjoy.

Finally, if you develop gestational diabetes in pregnancy, your dessert intake will look a little different. Do not despair. You will find the right foods in certain combinations that don't spike your blood sugar. Dessert is not off the table, but you will become a master at learning what works for your body and what doesn't.

SNACKS AND MINI MEALS

When you become pregnant, there's no slow roll into hunger any-more. You're not hungry, and then you're *starving*. There are many options, both prepackaged and DIY, that you can eat anytime during pregnancy, and that will be especially supportive if and when you're nursing.

SAVORY

- Crackers (nothing with added sugar or too many ingredients) dipped in full-fat, whole milk cottage cheese

- Frittata slice (see page 193)

- Hard-boiled eggs and fresh fruit

- Roasted sweet potatoes or roasted carrots dipped in two tablespoons of tahini

- Avocado mashed on toast, topped with hempseed hearts or pumpkin seeds and salt and pepper to taste

- Half an avocado stuffed with one-third of a cup of sauerkraut or two tablespoons of carrot-ginger dressing

- Half an avocado, mashed, with lemon juice and fine sea salt; use endive spears or another veggie of choice (or crackers) for dipping

- Avocado and egg salad (half an avocado mashed with two chopped hard-boiled eggs, seasoned to taste with salt and pepper); optional to serve with high-fiber crackers or one piece of toast

- Two eggs, any style (cooked with one tablespoon of grass-fed butter or olive oil) with high-fiber crackers or one piece of toast

- Two scrambled eggs with crumbled goat or feta cheese

- One to two cups of lentil vegetable soup (see page 255)

- One to two cups of butternut squash soup (see page 223) topped with pumpkin seeds or roasted chickpeas

- Seaweed snacks topped with hummus
- Ginger slaw with added cashews and optional protein like shredded chicken or tofu
- One to two ounces of cheddar cheese with one cup of grapes or sliced apples
- Caprese (sliced tomato and mozzarella with a drizzle of olive oil and optional balsamic vinegar)
- Watermelon and cucumber salad with feta cheese
- Quesadilla (wraps with cheddar cheese, sautéed spinach, and optional beans)
- Sardines (any way you like them)
- Everything Bagel Popcorn (page 220) with nuts or seeds of choice

SWEET

- One piece of Tahini Banana Bread (page 209)
- Baked oatmeal (see page 266) topped with full-fat plain Greek yogurt or nut butter
- Mixed fruit of choice (about one cup) topped with unsweetened coconut yogurt or full-fat plain Greek yogurt, cacao nibs, and chia seeds or hempseed hearts or a few tablespoons of granola
- An apple with nut butter of choice or tahini, as is or on top of toast or high-fiber crackers
- Smoothies (see page 191)
- Two Medjool dates stuffed with one to two tablespoons of nut butter, topped with a couple of chocolate chips and flaky sea salt
- Two Medjool dates stuffed with two tablespoons of goat cheese, topped with crushed pistachios

- Carrot Cake Muffins (page 206) topped with one tablespoon of grass-fed butter or nut butter
- Broiled grapefruit (broiled for five to eight minutes, flesh side up, with a drizzle of maple syrup and cinnamon), plus one fourth of a cup of shelled pistachios
- Energy Bites (page 261)
- High-fiber crackers topped with peanut butter, unsweetened shredded coconut, and a few dried cherries
- Avocado Chocolate Mousse (page 269)

CHAPTER 6

FOOD-RELATED COMPLAINTS
AND SIDE EFFECTS

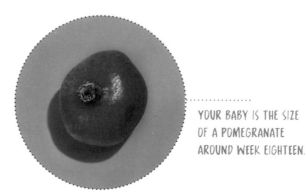

YOUR BABY IS THE SIZE
OF A POMEGRANATE
AROUND WEEK EIGHTEEN.

In the second trimester, in particular, food can be satisfying, comforting, and healing, but meals can also come with baggage, side effects, and tests that change the way you eat or think about food. Now that you have a full set of nutritional ninja skills, though, you can rest on that strong foundation when you deal with all the not-so-fun stuff. Don't worry, you've already gotten through the roughest patch. You're a pro. With high-quality foods, the right nutrients, meals and snacks that keep your blood sugar stable and curb your cravings, and a focus on self-care, you can handle anything that comes your way.

WEIGHT GAIN

I've found that weight gain is one of the hardest and most delicate topics—if not the hardest topic—for many pregnant women. Your shifting tastes, cravings, habits, and physiology may leave you feeling out of control, and people are starting to make comments about your body and your bump. No matter how seemingly innocent, unsolicited remarks about how you look—especially when you're bigger than you used to be—can trigger a reaction.

I get it. Sometimes your pregnant body doesn't fit what you dreamed a pregnant version of yourself would look and feel like. You may have fears about what's going to happen after pregnancy. Will you go back to looking the way you did before? First, and this is paramount, know that anxiety about weight gain is perfectly normal, and everyone handles it differently. Give yourself the space and freedom to have those thoughts, and it's okay to mourn your old body too. Don't keep it in. If there is not someone in your immediate circle you can talk to, there are a ton of resources to offer that helpful ear. If you feel depressed or if negative thoughts about your body occupy too much of your time, talk to someone on your health-care team ASAP.

Let's talk about the factors that are going into your weight gain, because as complex as these feelings may be, understanding the biology behind it may (I hope) give you a sense of wonder about it too. It doesn't come down to eating larger portions, or even that there is literally another person inside of you. It starts with some pretty remarkable changes in the physiology of your body. As I've discussed, in pregnancy, your blood volume *increases*. Your breast tissue grows. In addition to the baby, you're carrying a placenta and a uterus full of amniotic fluid. Even if you don't eat an ounce more than usual, your body will add pounds—for some quickly and for others more slowly.

PREGNANCY WEIGHT GAIN (APPROXIMATE VALUES)

· Maternal breast tissue: two pounds

· Baby: seven to eight pounds

· Placenta: one to two pounds

· Uterus: two pounds

· Fat, protein, and nutrient stores: seven pounds

· Amniotic fluid: two pounds

· Maternal blood: four pounds

· Bodily fluids: four pounds

Total: twenty-five to thirty-five pounds

While I never want you to fixate on a number, you're probably wondering how much weight you "should" be gaining. Since all humans are different, there is no right answer. You might have seen in your ferocious online sleuthing that the CDC and the American College of Obstetricians and Gynecologists (ACOG) have recommendations for pregnancy based on body mass index, or BMI (a measure of body fat based on height and weight). I've provided a link to the chart in the resources section (see page 275). That said, BMI is not something I've ever counseled a woman to follow, because it doesn't take a multitude of factors into account. For example, if going by BMI, many professional athletes would rank as obese.

Weight gain is also inconsistent during pregnancy, meaning it's not the same week to week. The average weight gain while carrying a single baby, according to the ACOG, is anywhere from one to five pounds in the first trimester and half a pound to one pound a week in the second and third trimesters. However, I've seen women gain a lot of weight in the beginning and others in the final months. Some weeks you won't see any weight gain (especially if you are nauseated or unable to keep food down), while other weeks you may pack on the pounds. Your baby also experiences growth spurts, and your hormones and appetite fluctuate.

In short, please don't obsess about the number on the scale. Most of the time, there is absolutely nothing wrong—as long as you bear the following in mind.

- If you find that you have gained five pounds or more in a week and are experiencing swelling and water retention, reach out to your medical team as it could be a sign of something more serious like preeclampsia.

- If you are especially worried or anxious about your weight gain or have a negative relationship with the scale, my recommendation is not to weigh yourself at home. If you don't want to see the number at your doctor's office, let the nurse and your OB know. Ask to be weighed backward or close your eyes when getting weighed. If there is cause for concern, they will let you know.

Finally, know that a healthy pregnancy is one that supports a healthy baby and mom, and the numbers on the scale don't tell us much about nutrition and health. If you are consuming a healthy diet, meaning one that nourishes you and your baby, and your provider is monitoring the growth and development of your baby and has no misgivings, then you are doing a top-notch job. Never forget that your body is changing for a reason, and that reason is nothing short of miraculous.

WHAT ABOUT THESE . . . STRETCH MARKS?!?

Stretch marks are often the result of rapid changes in weight, both gain and loss, and they typically appear on your belly, thighs, breasts, or hips. Normally, your skin adapts to continuous movement by expanding and contracting, but when you're pregnant, sometimes it doesn't have enough leeway. When the body grows faster than the skin covering it, the skin tears slightly, and the resulting scar is what we know as a stretch mark. The fact that you get stretch marks is mainly due to genetics, and while you can't fully prevent them, eating well and staying hydrated can help to minimize them. This can also help to slow the weight gain while keeping your skin supple and hydrated.

THE C WORD: CRAVINGS

Now that we have covered the foundations of second-trimester nutrition, let's talk about the peanut-butter-covered-fried-pickle-with-Nutella-on-top in the room. Cravings! You've heard about them, you've seen them on TV, and now you're about to live them. Not every woman is going to wake up in the middle of the night wanting to drink pickle juice out of the jar, but you will crave *something* (for me, it was roasted chicken and baked potatoes with butter . . . all the time), which will be a not-so-subtle hint that your body needs, well, *something*. In fact, pregnancy cravings may indicate that your body is deficient in certain nutrients. So if you feel the urge, check out the chart below to better translate this odd language your body is talking.

CRAVING	WHAT IT MAY MEAN
Dairy, especially cow's milk	You might need more calcium, but you also may need more iodine. Iodine needs in pregnancy increase by almost 50 percent compared to non-pregnancy, and milk is rich in it.
Carbs	These are the easiest things to keep down when you're not feeling well, so pay attention to what else might be causing your morning sickness or acid reflux. During the third trimester, you may also crave additional carbs because your body is building its fat stores.
Sugary foods	Sugar spikes your blood sugar, so needing a quick fix may simply indicate that you're hungry. Work to keep your blood sugar stable during the day by including protein, fat, and fiber with every meal and snack. Again, you also crave what you eat, so the more sugar you have, the more you want it. See more about blood-sugar control on page 133.

Fruit	You could be dehydrated or deficient in folate or vitamin C. Your needs for these nutrients go up in pregnancy, and fruit is chock-full.
Salty foods	Salt is essential for your baby's organ growth and the development of your uterine tissue, so this craving could mean you need more salt in your diet. Instead of reaching for potato chips, try eating olives, pickles, roasted chickpeas with a pinch of salt, or salted nuts or seeds of your choice. See page 221 for two delicious marinated cucumber recipes that will nip that salty, crunchy craving in the bud.

GET MOVING

Eating well during pregnancy is only part of the equation. I'm constantly asked about exercise too. The short answer is: do it. Exercise, specifically anything that gets your heart rate up, has a ton of benefits, including reducing the risk of gestational diabetes, preeclampsia, and cesarean birth. It helps with constipation, minimizes back pain, controls blood sugar, and boosts your mental health while reducing stress and depression. It can keep you within a healthy weight range during pregnancy and help your body recover faster after.

If you have concerns about modifying your workouts or how much aerobic activity is too much, talk to your provider. I had those questions and concerns too. Getting pregnant was a long journey for me, and I was nervous about doing anything that would jeopardize it. I also had one exercise instructor tell me not to jump while pregnant, which terrified me! So, I didn't, and then a million people told me afterward that my instructor was 100 percent wrong.

Your doctor is likely to clear you for cardio, but they may not offer specifics. Listen to your body; take it easy at first and slowly work up to more movement, especially if you're not normally a big exerciser. Base your workouts on your fitness level pre-pregnancy, and take advantage of the many online classes for pregnant women. If you go to a group class, share how far along you are with your instructor so they can offer adjustments or modifications and watch you closely.

Don't underestimate the benefits of a vigorous walk either. We often feel that if we aren't pouring sweat, we aren't getting an effective workout, but that couldn't be further from the truth. Divvy up your workouts however you like, from five thirty-minute workouts a week to ten-minute chunks whenever you have the time.

Your motivation and interests will ebb and flow, so don't be hard on yourself. When you are nauseated and exhausted in the first trimester, then large and uncomfortable in any position during the third trimester, remember that you can always adjust and try something new. Your goal is to get your blood flowing, keep your energy up, and connect with yourself and your baby.

GASTROINTESTINAL ISSUES

During your second trimester, your progesterone levels are still on the rise. This means you may notice even more GI issues, like gas, constipation, and bloating. Because you have a little (or big) bump, though, your bloating may be invisible to everyone but you. Regardless, if you didn't experience constipation in your first trimester and skimmed over chapter 3, let's revisit it, shall we?

If you are constipated, try the following:

· **Increase naturally fiber-rich foods like vegetables, especially leafy green ones like kale and spinach:** When I was pregnant, I ate a kale salad (see page 230) at least twice a week, and this wasn't just because I liked it so much. (It also helped me go to the bathroom.)

· **Eat beans and/or seeds:** Incorporate beans into your regular meal rotation unless you become too gassy. For seeds, like chia or ground flax, just two tablespoons provide six grams of fiber. Add them to smoothies, baked goods, and oatmeal.

· **Hydrate:** You need adequate water to move all that fiber along, roughly one hundred ounces a day. Otherwise, you will have all the bloat without any relief.

- **Consider a magnesium supplement:** Magnesium citrate or glycinate can ease things along—refer to page 35 for more information. Start on the lower end of the recommended dosage and slowly build up to a maximum of five hundred milligrams per day.

ACID REFLUX

The burning pressure you might feel in your chest has to do with a hormone called relaxin. Relaxin's purpose is to soften the ligaments, joints, and, in the third trimester, the cervix to prepare your body for childbirth. But it also relaxes the sphincter muscle at the base of your esophagus, which may cause acid from your stomach to bubble up. Couple that with the fact that your baby is growing and putting pressure on all your organs, and you've got heartburn.

Acid reflux can happen at any point in pregnancy, but many people start to notice it in the second trimester. Here are some things that can help.

- **Try to understand the cause of your acid reflux:** Is it because of a specific acidic food or beverage? Are you eating too much at one time? Are you eating too late into the evening or going too long without food? Once you get a handle on what your food trigger(s) might be, you can make modifications.

- **Limit certain foods:** Common culprits include citrus fruits (oranges, grapefruits, lemons), tomatoes and tomato sauce, chocolate (I'm sorry, this one is hard for me to accept too), spicy foods, fried foods, garlic and raw onions (leeks and shallots may be tolerated better), dairy, coffee, and carbonated beverages. Limiting or eliminating these foods may alleviate your acid reflux. You may find that having dairy a few days a week is fine but daily worsens your symptoms, or you may have to cut out the cheese altogether. Keeping a food journal to track what you're eating, rather than relying on your memory when you have so much else going on, can narrow in on the culprit.

- **Eat smaller meals more frequently:** Reducing portions and eating more mini meals throughout the day may offer relief (see the snack ideas on page 115). But that doesn't mean eating constantly. The goal is to feel satisfied for at least two hours after a meal without pushing the time between meals for too long, which can lead to more stomach acid. You'll find the right balance.

· **Exercise:** After meals, go for a walk or do light exercise that keeps you upright. Moving around supports digestion and controls blood sugar.

· **Eat dinner at least two hours before you go to bed**—and chew slowly.

· **Limit antacids:** Try to hold off on taking antacids, as they can interfere with the absorption of nutrients and start a negative cycle of tummy issues. They also disrupt your microbiome because they destroy some of your stomach acid, which allows unhealthy bacteria to flourish. But you know your body best; if you are in tremendous discomfort and know that antacids will help, it's okay to find the relief you need.

URINARY TRACT INFECTIONS (UTIS)

UTIs are common during pregnancy because, as your uterus expands, it puts pressure on the bladder, which then never fully empties. The longer urine stays in your bladder, the more bacteria grow and multiply, and this can lead to UTIs. Stay hydrated so that your bladder is regularly flushing itself out, and urinate as soon as you feel the urge. I know you are running to the bathroom a lot already, but trust me, it's worth it to stay on top of this one.

There is research that suggests that drinking unsweetened cranberry juice can reduce the risk of developing a UTI by up to 35 percent. If you have a UTI or are prone to them, drink a cup or eight ounces a day. Kefir has also been shown to prevent *E. coli*—the bacteria that can cause UTIs—from "sticking" to the urinary tract wall, and since it is fermented, it has plenty of other benefits.

Finally, bad bacteria loves sugar, so aim to reduce your intake.

LEG CRAMPS

About half of you reading this book—meaning 50 percent of all pregnant women—will get leg cramps during pregnancy. The best way to describe them is a sudden, painful tightening or spasm in your calf and/or foot. They are usually brief but can hurt a lot. In the moment, the best way to relieve them is to stretch your calf by flexing your foot and pulling it back with your hand toward your body. Doctors and researchers don't know what causes leg cramps, but they could be related to a deficiency in magnesium or calcium or B vitamins, dehydration, changes in circulation, sitting for too long, or exercising too much.

If you have frequent leg cramps, you should chat with your OB. Some women also get relief from eating foods rich in magnesium, calcium, and vitamin B (see the chart on page 16 for your best food sources). You can also take a magnesium supplement, specifically the glycinate form, but nutrition should be your first stop. I don't recommend you take an additional calcium supplement separate from your prenatal, but instead, rely on food-based calcium sources. Finally, aim for daily walks (fifteen to twenty minutes) as well as elevating your legs on a chair or on a few stacked pillows when you lie down.

ANXIETY

Some pregnant women develop anxiety beyond what they felt pre-pregnancy. This may be caused by fluctuating hormones, sleep disturbances, and a general sense that life is about to dramatically change. If you notice a shift in your mood that is significant enough to affect your daily life, please, please don't keep it in. Reach out to your OB, therapist, partner, best friend—anyone who can be empathetic and help you find a path to get support. Sometimes, you may need medication for anxiety, which is a call you and your doctor can make.

Research shows that lower levels of vitamin D are associated with a host of mental challenges, including anxiety, so try to get out into the sun during the day for at least thirty minutes and make sure your prenatal contains sufficient vitamin D (see page 32 to determine your optimal level). Foods rich in zinc have also been shown to reduce anxiety, and magnesium (in the glycinate form) can calm your nervous system, especially before bed.

INSOMNIA

Why? Because of all the symptoms we just discussed! Between the acid reflux, congestion, leg cramps, and anxiety, it's no wonder that sleep can become tougher in the second and third trimesters. As with most things, good nutrition can help. Consider magnesium to wind down before bed, and eat nuts like almonds, walnuts, pistachios, and cashews, which are rich in zinc, magnesium, and melatonin, a naturally produced hormone that regulates the sleep-wake cycle. The fat in nuts may also prevent middle-of-the-night blood-sugar dips (which could wake you up). Some people may also benefit from a small nighttime snack:

- Pumpkin seeds plus one tablespoon of unsweetened dried cherries

- A few crackers with one tablespoon of nut or seed butter

- A banana with a handful of almonds or cashews

Just as adding in supportive foods and practices can help with sleep, you may also want to cut some things out. Caffeine can stay in your system for up to ten hours, so if you have your last cup of coffee at 12 p.m., when 10 p.m. rolls around, it may still be keeping you from falling asleep and affecting the quality of your sleep. Blue light from electronics like your phone or TV reduces melatonin production, so be sure to turn them off at least thirty minutes before bed, and don't check your emails in the middle of the night (been there, done that at three in the morning).

HEADACHES AND MIGRAINES

In the second trimester, some women suffer from more headaches and migraines than they did before they were pregnant. While this is often due to changes in hormones, weight, and blood volume, it can also be from stress, constipation, dehydration, fatigue, or mineral deficiencies (often iron and calcium). Headaches are also a side effect of constipation; on the flip side, having regular bowel movements can decrease your headaches.

Severe headaches that begin suddenly after month six can indicate preeclampsia. If this is the case, or if your headaches or migraines are debilitating, contact your doctor.

Luckily, most of the time headaches are treatable at home. Pay attention to the following:

· **Hydration:** Here I go again. Make sure you're drinking enough water every day (one hundred ounces), especially in the morning. Dehydration can lead to headaches and/or migraines. And remember, it's not just water that can hydrate you (see page 61).

· **Magnesium:** If you aren't already taking a magnesium supplement, now may be a good time to start. Try one hundred milligrams of magnesium glycinate and gradually increase that amount if your symptoms aren't subsiding. Most pregnant women should be taking between three hundred and five hundred milligrams of magnesium a day, and while you can get a lot from food, supplementing offers extra support.

· **Vitamin B$_{12}$:** A deficiency of vitamin B$_{12}$ has been linked to neurological problems, including headaches, so make sure you're getting enough from your food intake (see the chart on page 17 for options) as well as getting tested for a possible deficiency.

Finally, focus on getting enough sleep and exercise, as a lack of either can contribute to headaches. I know it can be hard to find time to de-stress, but that little bit of self-care will pay huge dividends.

GESTATIONAL DIABETES

According to the CDC, gestational diabetes is a condition that 2 to 10 percent of pregnant women get. You'll almost certainly be tested for it.

Gestational diabetes (GD) occurs when too much glucose (sugar) remains in the blood during pregnancy instead of being metabolized for energy. If it's untreated, you're at greater risk for preeclampsia and difficulties giving birth, both because of longer labor time and a larger-than-average birth weight for the baby. Babies born to mothers with GD are at risk for metabolic syndrome, obesity, and diabetes. That's the bad news. The overwhelmingly good news is that GD can easily be controlled with diet and exercise, and it usually goes away after the birth.

Your blood sugar is regulated by a hormone called insulin, which is secreted by your pancreas. When you're pregnant, your insulin levels increase because insulin fosters tissue growth for you and your baby. For some women, certain pregnancy hormones disrupt insulin production, which means that you don't have enough insulin to lower your blood sugar to an appropriate level. When your blood sugar goes up and stays up, you get a diagnosis of gestational diabetes.

Again, most pregnant women won't develop GD, but certain risk factors contribute to it, including being overweight, not getting enough exercise, having high blood pressure or heart disease, having polycystic ovarian syndrome (PCOS), or having had GD or a baby over nine pounds during a previous pregnancy.

Testing for Gestational Diabetes

Lab tests are never fun, but you'll get through them by remembering that the goal here is to act proactively versus reactively. Nine out of ten of my clients don't know much about what to expect and how to prepare. Let's fix that.

Testing for GD usually happens in the second trimester, anywhere from week twenty-four to twenty-eight. In some practices, older moms (hi, my name is Stephanie, and I was an older mom!) will be tested as early as sixteen weeks (and possibly again later), since studies show that their bodies may become resistant to insulin earlier than moms under thirty-five. Your first screening— called the glucose screening test or glucose challenge test—is a one-hour test that measures how your body responds to sugar. An hour before your test, you'll drink a sugary beverage (fifty grams of glucose) called glucola, then have your blood drawn. Warning: the drink tastes like off-brand Gatorade with the consistency of maple syrup, and some pregnant women get nause-ated or headaches from it, especially if they are not used to having that much sugar in one sitting. Also, some women who follow a low-carb diet might get a false positive because their body isn't used to processing this much sugar at once. If that may be you, either increase your carb intake the week before the test or talk to your OB about skipping it. If you don't have any risk factors for GD, there are options for monitoring your blood sugar at home instead. The test differs from practice to practice, so have a conversation with your health-care team about what to expect.

For a better experience, here are a few tips:

· Ask for lemon- or lime-flavored glucola, as it contains less food dye than the fruit punch or orange flavors.

· Ask for it cold, as it improves the taste (sort of).

· Eat before the test, even if it's first thing in the morning. *This is not a fasting test!* I, as well as many clients and friends, was told to fast beforehand, and it simply has no scientific backing. Aim to have a high-protein, high-fat meal (e.g., eggs and avocado, yogurt and nuts) before you go, as fat and protein slow the absorption of sugar. This will make you feel better and give a more accurate outcome.

You may have heard of alternatives, like a jelly bean test or juice test, but these aren't accurate or reliable, so I don't recommend them. However, there is at least one organic test free of dyes, additives, and artificial flavoring on the market that may be more pleasant for some of you. I wish I had known about this when I was pregnant. If you have concerns about the traditional test, talk with your care team ahead of your test date to ensure you can use it. Finally, there are ways to monitor your sugars at home, so if you aren't at high risk for GD and don't want to drink the drink, talk to your provider about this option.

If you "fail" this test (as I did, probably because I had been told to fast—and I'm still angry about it!), then you will likely have to schedule a follow-up three-hour test. For this test, you *do* fast beforehand and have your blood sugar measured. Then you drink one hundred grams of glucose and get tested at one, two, and three hours. Pack a meal to eat as soon as your time is up because you will be starving. As with test number one, some women opt out and choose instead to monitor their blood sugar at home. If you choose to take this route, talk to your health-care team, as there are options on how to do this. If you fail your second blood glucose test and are diagnosed with gestational diabetes, *do not worry*. You will be connected with a diabetes educator or registered dietitian to learn how to navigate an appropriate diet and keep GD in check and how to track your blood sugar at home. It may feel terrifying and like a lot more work, especially at first, but you will get the hang of it. Once you are able to maintain normal blood glucose levels, you and your baby will be A-OK. I highly recommend the book by Lily Nichols, RDN, CDE, CLT, *Real Food for Gestational Diabetes*, as an invaluable resource.

Balancing Your Blood Sugar (Whether or Not You Have GD)

Even if you pass the first and/or second glucose tolerance test and are not diagnosed with gestational diabetes, blood sugar control is still essential. First,
your blood sugar influences your energy and appetite throughout the day.
With balanced levels, you are less likely to experience energy and mood
crashes. Second, understanding your blood sugar sets you up for more struc-
tured eating (as opposed to grazing—or ravenously scarfing). You'll know
when to eat to feel full and energetic, and how much. You'll be in control of
your eating and hunger rather than letting your eating and hunger control you.

To balance your blood sugar, do the following:

· **Eat consistently:** Think three meals a day plus one to three snacks.

· **Include a protein source with every meal and snack:** For
example, if you have an apple, pair it with nut butter, cheese, or hummus.

· **Eat fats:** Fat can decrease the amount of insulin produced in response to
a higher-carb meal. Fats also keep us fuller for a longer period of time, so
we're less tempted to reach for carb-heavy or sugary snacks. Also, fat
simply makes food taste better. Fat for the win!

- **Eat a breakfast that contains protein:** When you wake up, your body is in a fasted state, so it's far more sensitive to the food you eat. Therefore, the longer you go without eating, the more likely you are to have a glucose spike when you *do*. Be sure your breakfast includes protein and fat to fill you up.

- **Aim to reduce refined sugar:** This will help prevent blood sugar spikes and crashes. You're only human, though, and humans like sugar, so if and when you eat something sweet, try to do it after a meal that contains protein, fat, and fiber. That combo will reduce the spike. I am a huge proponent of enjoying your food, but we do tend to crave what we eat, meaning that when it comes to sugar, it's a self-fulfilling cycle. (Also, "desserts" is "stressed" spelled backward.) Just sayin'.

- **Hydrate:** We often reach for food when, in fact, we are dehydrated.

- **Watch the coffee:** Caffeine can contribute to a crash (what goes up must come down), and when we crash, we often look for an upper, like sugar or more caffeine. Additionally, a lot of us connect having sugar with enjoying a cup of coffee, so it can be a double whammy.

- **Move:** Aim for a walk after meals. Even a short one will work to control blood sugar.

- **Get those z's:** When we're tired, we look for foods that give us quick energy, like sugar and excess carbs. A lack of sleep also contributes to insulin sensitivity, meaning a higher likelihood of developing diabetes.

BLOOD SUGAR AND ARTIFICIAL SWEETENERS

Artificial sweeteners are a lot sweeter than natural sugars, which can make your palate expect and need a higher level of sweetness to feel satisfied. Studies also show that certain artificial sweeteners have the same or a *more* negative impact on blood sugar levels than natural sugar, and they decimate the beneficial bacteria in our gut. Even sweeteners that don't affect blood sugar—like stevia, monk fruit, allulose, and erythritol—still exacerbate your sweet tooth, so although they are considered safe in pregnancy, I still recommend limiting them, or better yet, removing them entirely.

If you want to work in less-sweet versions of your favorite treats (like drinking your morning coffee without sugar), know that your taste buds will adjust—usually in about two weeks—so you won't hate me for long.

GESTATIONAL HYPERTENSION AND PREECLAMPSIA

Gestational hypertension is high blood pressure during pregnancy. This condition occurs in about three out of every fifty pregnancies, and it's typically diagnosed around week twenty. While it's not known what causes this condition, women who have had high blood pressure before pregnancy, have diabetes or kidney disease, are pregnant with multiples, are under twenty or over forty, or were overweight before pregnancy are more at risk.

Preeclampsia is similar to gestational hypertension in that they're both diagnosed around the same time, based mostly on elevated blood pressure readings, and gestational hypertension can lead to preeclampsia. But preeclampsia is more serious because it's marked by protein in the urine, which indicates that the kidneys are malfunctioning. Preeclampsia is also rarer—only about one in twenty-five women develop it—but it can lead to issues including placental abruption (when the placenta pulls away from the uterus), low birth weight, or—at its worst—eclampsia, which causes seizures.

The good news is that gestational hypertension usually goes away after birth, and preeclampsia is treatable, thanks to modern medicine. There is also so much you can do at home using—you guessed it—proper nutrition. If you have or are worried about gestational hypertension or preeclampsia, in addition to eating the most nutrient-dense, fresh, whole foods you can find, focus on the following:

- **Magnesium:** Not only is magnesium a frontline medical treatment prescribed by doctors to treat preeclampsia and eclampsia, but foods rich in magnesium can balance blood pressure.

- **Potassium:** This electrolyte lowers blood pressure, so be sure to eat potassium-rich foods, including bananas, butternut squash, kidney and black beans, peas, avocados, potatoes, apricots, cucumbers, sweet potatoes, spinach, watermelon, pomegranates, and coconut water.

- **Calcium:** Preeclampsia is associated with poor calcium metabolism, and studies show that having enough calcium in your diet (and prenatal) lowers your risk.

- **Protein:** Women who don't eat enough protein during pregnancy are more at risk of developing hypertension and preeclampsia.

- **Sodium:** You might assume that if you eat less sodium during pregnancy, you'll lower your risk of hypertension and preeclampsia. But this isn't the case. Sodium is essential during pregnancy, especially when it comes to maintaining steady blood pressure. Look for whole foods that contain sodium, like pickles, olives, or cheeses, or add your own high-quality variety to your meals.

- **Vitamins C, D, and E:** Make sure you're getting adequate time in the sun every day, and load up on foods rich in these essential vitamins.

Flip back to page 16 for a list of all the foods you can incorporate to get these vitamins and nutrients.

I hope you don't have to battle any of the side effects I've described here, but if you do, food can help, and food can heal. Someone once told me that the only cure for a pregnancy-related complication is giving birth, but that's only half the story. Good nutrition can work wonders too. Let it perform its magic for you—and your baby.

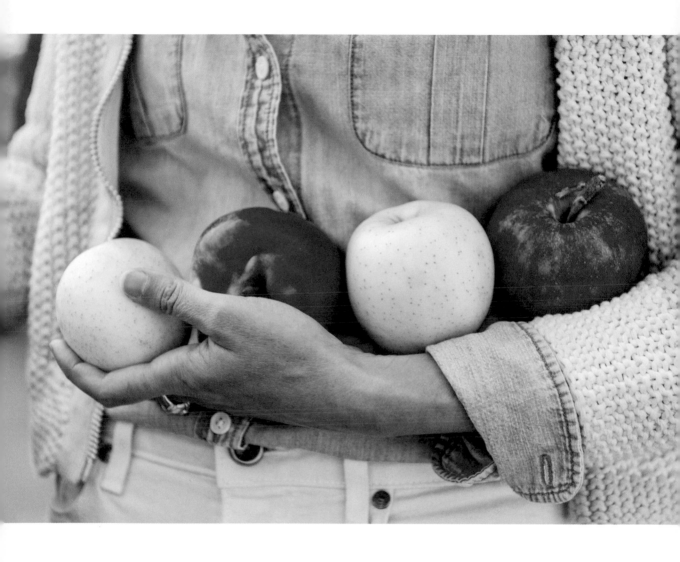

SECTION THREE: THE THIRD TRIMESTER

A-l-m-o-s-t there. Yep, all that hard work, dedication, and endurance is about to pay off. Though it may still feel like an eternity, in just a few short months, you'll finally get to meet this beautiful creature you've been so dutifully caring for (and eating for) since day one.

While you're busy setting up the nursery and installing the car seat, it's also time to prepare your body for birth and recovery. In this section, we'll start with the nutritional foundation for the third trimester because, while by now you're hopefully in a healthful, nourishing relationship with food and nutrition, there are some new challenges in the final stretch. You'll want to ensure you're fortified with the right nutrients for your baby to get yourself over any last bumps in the road and to set the stage for an uncomplicated childbirth and recovery. You have so much to prepare for, and you're about to be a busy (and tired) mama bear taking care of your new cub, so let's make sure you have everything you need. There's tremendous joy in welcoming your baby; let's make food a part of it.

CHAPTER 7

NUTRITIONAL NEEDS AND
THIRD TRIMESTER CHANGES

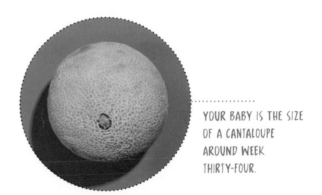

YOUR BABY IS THE SIZE
OF A CANTALOUPE
AROUND WEEK
THIRTY-FOUR.

Your little one is making their presence known. Not only are their lungs developing, eyes opening, and red blood cells forming, but they're also getting big—like, really big. Some of their movements—like an elbow pressed into your bladder or kicks to your ribs—may be getting a little less cute than those hiccups were a month or two ago. You might have traded your maternity pillow for the couch (or anywhere that is actually comfortable), and you probably fill up quickly and have to urinate *constantly*. And the swelling . . .

Some people will do well just continuing the dietary course they've established, but a few minor tweaks can make that third-trimester sprint to the finish even more seamless. Baby is having their last growth and developmental spurt (think elbows—you'll feel them!), so let's make sure you both get what you need.

NUTRITION IN THE THIRD TRIMESTER

First and foremost, continue to take your prenatal vitamins. Many women assume that prenatals are just for the first and second trimesters when a baby's bones and organs are doing their main developing, but the vitamins and minerals in prenatals are for your benefit too. You need vitamin C for your immune system and D_3 for strong bones, not to mention iodine for your thyroid and magnesium for your heart and brain. (Turn to the prenatal chart on page 30 for a quick refresher.)

In addition to all the good stuff found in prenatals, women in their third trimester need to pay attention to protein, iron, and probiotics. Here's why:

Protein

Protein needs are the highest now. Most women need around one hundred grams of protein a day in the third trimester, which is a full twenty grams more than in the first. Sixty-seven percent of pregnant women don't hit that goal, so let's underline that point: *It's time to eat a lot of protein-rich foods.*

Why so much protein? First, it keeps you satisfied, helps to prevent blood sugar dips and spikes, and keeps you energized. It also helps prevent swelling and supports your vascular system with all the extra blood that's flowing through your veins. Protein-rich foods also tend to contain other nutrients needed during pregnancy, like iron, zinc, choline, and vitamin B_{12}.

In the third trimester, it can be hard to know when to eat because you don't get hungry as often, and you fill up fast. Just focus—as you have been—on trying to get in a protein source with every meal and snack. Also, at this stage Bone Broth (page 247) comes in very handy; sipping your protein is easy, enjoyable, and soothing at a time when you need all the pampering you can get. Plus, bone broth provides much-needed hydration and electrolytes.

Aim to get your protein from a combination of animal- and plant-based sources. In addition to bone broth, here are my favorites:

· Eggs (ideally pasture-raised)

- Fish and seafood (ideally wild caught)

- Beef, lamb, pork, and game meat like bison or venison (ideally from pasture-raised animals)

- Poultry like chicken and turkey (ideally from pasture-raised birds)

- Dairy sources like cheese (ideally from grass-fed or pasture-raised animals) and yogurt (plain and full fat)

- Nuts/nut butter and seeds

- Legumes, including beans, lentils, and peas

Iron

I discussed iron earlier and why it's so important. But the third trimester is a whole new ball game. Remember how your blood volume increases by 50 percent? Well, now it's going up even more and your iron intake needs to keep pace.

You should have your iron levels tested at the start of pregnancy and before entering your third trimester. Anemia is common in pregnancy and can happen at any time, but it's most likely to crop up in the second and third trimesters. Maternal anemia can increase the risk of low birth weight and is associated with delayed neurocognitive development. Symptoms include feeling tired and weak, becoming especially pale, a rapid heartbeat or heart palpitations, shortness of breath, and the inability to maintain body warmth. Risk factors include having had anemia before, having two pregnancies close together, being pregnant with more than one child, not consuming enough iron (especially animal protein), and frequently exercising or training vigorously. If you have any of these symptoms or fall into any of the risk categories, ask your doctor to test your iron, especially if it hasn't been tested recently.

If you are anemic, or if you become anemic, consider an iron supplement. Look for "iron bisglycinate" on the label, because it is better absorbed and easier on the stomach. You can also look into a desiccated liver supplement. Try not to take your iron supplement at the same time you consume anything with calcium, since calcium can decrease its absorption.

Again, there are two forms of iron in food: heme and nonheme. Plants and plant-based protein only contain nonheme, while animal-based protein contains heme. While I love beans, lentils, peas, and other plant-based sources for their overall nutritional benefits, only a small amount (2 to 13 percent) of that iron gets absorbed by your body. Foods rich in vitamin C support the absorption of nonheme iron, so if you lean in the plant-based direction, consider including foods like tomatoes, peppers, and citrus with your meals and cooking in a cast-iron skillet.

Heme iron, on the other hand, is easily absorbed by your body, up to 40 percent. Opt for beef, lamb, game meat, organ meat, and to a lesser degree, eggs and shellfish.

Finally, you'll want to keep up your iron stores once the baby is born, but I'll talk more about that in chapter 9.

Probiotics

In chapter 2, I discussed the importance of probiotics in pregnancy, but they serve a special role in the third trimester; for one, they can reduce the chance of developing preeclampsia.

Because an ounce of prevention is worth a pound of cure, if you have a C-section, whether planned or not, or if you or your baby received antibiotics during childbirth, give the child an infant probiotic. The birth canal is full of microorganisms that populate a baby's microbiome, and without this initial exposure, C-section babies are more likely to develop chronic immune-related conditions like eczema, allergies, celiac disease, and even diabetes.

Foods rich in probiotics include kefir, yogurt (including dairy-free varieties), certain cottage cheeses, and fermented veggies including kimchi and miso, so eat all of them with abandon (unless you find that they upset your stomach, in which case start slow and/or opt for nondairy varieties). You can also take a probiotic supplement.

YOUR BODY IN THE THIRD TRIMESTER

You've been through this twice before: massive changes to your physical, emotional, and physiological self. Just when you think you've gotten used to your new body, *bam!* it shifts again. You may be swollen all over, and you may not remember what your feet look like (are they even down there?), yet you also have the most glorious hair of your life *and* a head-to-toe glow. Your third-trimester body is a beautiful thing, so let's walk through some of what it's going through.

Appetite Changes

By now, your uterus has gotten so large that it is compressing your stomach. This lack of space can make eating large meals a no-go, and you may notice you get full easily, then hungry soon after. You may also find that you can't eat half of what's on your plate, so you save it for later (I call this "later food").

Snacks become a *must* during the third trimester, so consult chapter 5 for what to eat and how to time them. Rest assured that if you feel the need to graze all day, with only thirty minutes or so between snacks, that's completely okay. Remember to pair a protein and a fiber so you're getting as much nutrition as you can and not filling up on food that won't leave you satisfied.

SWELLING

During the third trimester, your body retains more water with each passing day. The extra fluids in your tissues make you a little softer all over (like a giant waterbed), which allows you to expand as your baby grows. This fluid also loosens your pelvic joints, paving the way for delivery.

If you haven't yet cut out processed snacks and meals or fast food, now is the time. The chemicals and additives can damage your gut and cause inflammation. Also, keep hydrating. It may seem counterintuitive, but drinking more water moves the fluid in your tissues out into your bloodstream and through your kidneys. Aim for at least one hundred ounces (or at least eight cups) of water (or other hydrating beverages/foods; see page 61) per day. As a bonus, staying hydrated can prevent preterm labor.

Keep up with your electrolytes too, which maintain fluid balance.

Some foods are natural diuretics, meaning they move water out of your tissues and into your kidneys so you can excrete more urine (and hopefully make that swelling go down). These include asparagus, cucumbers, celery, beets, pineapple, watermelon, and grapes.

Other ways to alleviate puffy ankles and feet include the following:

- Lying on your back and putting your legs up against a wall, feet pointed toward the ceiling, or lying on your back with your feet and ankles elevated on pillows
- Walking, even just ten to fifteen minutes, to get the blood moving
- Wearing compression socks. These may take twelve to fourteen days to reduce swelling, but ... aah ... sweet relief when they do.

Some degree of swelling in pregnancy is normal, but if you experience uneven swelling, confusion, extreme pain, dizziness, or headaches, call your doctor to confirm that it's not a symptom of an underlying condition.

CHAPTER 8

PREPARING FOR THE BIG DAY

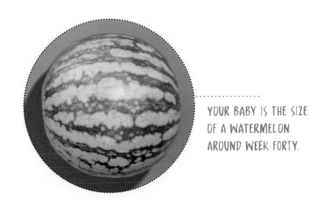

YOUR BABY IS THE SIZE
OF A WATERMELON
AROUND WEEK FORTY.

The final countdown has begun. Whether you're in week thirty-six or forty-two (oof), if it's your first baby or your fifth, know that you've done something miraculous. You've built and nurtured a person from scratch, taken care of their needs—and your own—and given the better part of yourself to make another human the best they can be. You are already a mom, which is the hardest, most amazing job in the world, and I want to congratulate you. Now, on to the big day.

By the end of the third trimester, many women are so busy thinking about their birth plan that they forget entirely about a food plan. The truth is that good nutrition will help with birth, labor, and recovery. When I had my son, I went in unprepared and regretted it, so learn from my mistakes. Food can fuel you during delivery and provide much-needed nutrition (there's a world beyond hospital Jell-O!). It will help heal you after you get home with your baby, too, and a little advance planning will ensure you have everything you need to feel nourished and supported.

THE NESTING PERIOD

In the weeks before your baby comes, you may feel the desire to organize your home, clean out closets, wash the dog, toss out old clothes, build shelves, bake banana bread, start your holiday card list . . . I'm tired just thinking about it! This is called the nesting period, and it's a normal hormonal response as your body and mind prepare for the arrival of your little one. In the third trimester, the hormones estrogen and estradiol peak, and with an additional rise in adrenaline, you suddenly have a surge of energy.

Now, you've probably given a lot of thought about how you are going to feed your baby, but what about you? Use the nesting period to prepare for your needs because mama has to eat too. Don't wait to stock your fridge and freezer until after the baby's born because by then life will be all about them. Think ahead while the crib's getting assembled and the toys are being put in place. Spending a few hours on assembling your food and nutrition plan will pay significant dividends.

Here are some things to think about to make this easier on you and your family:

- **Cook meals to freeze, which will last six months in the freezer:** In the recipe section, I have included some of my favorite meals to make ahead of time that freeze well and are nurturing and satisfying. Think stews, lasagna, meatballs, broth, etc.

- **Meal delivery:** A lot of women find it helpful to schedule deliveries in advance with a service (if that's an option where you live). Or plan to order from local restaurants. You can also ask friends or family members to set up a meal train to either drop off or order meals for you. Don't be afraid to ask—they want to help, and this is an easy way to make your loved ones feel like they are contributing.

· **Grocery delivery:** Look into ordering your groceries online. I quickly found out that schlepping groceries, a stroller, a car seat, and a baby is no picnic, and this option was a real lifesaver.

THE FREEZER IS YOUR FRIEND

I am a huge fan of the freezer. You can stock up on healthy, nutritious fruits and vegetables and bag and freeze them or cook your comfort foods ahead of time to save for later. Some people have concerns about freezing food or are out of the habit, so here are my guidelines, pointers, and tips:

· Is freezing healthy? Absolutely! As long as it's done properly, it locks in nutrients and freshness so your items are just as healthy as the day they went into the freezer.

· You may have heard not to use glass, which can shatter when liquid expands. I'm fine with glass for recipes that will be thawed or reheated in the microwave (as long as you're cautious about overfilling). For recipes that you won't reheat in their container, like bars or cookies, I like to use silicone bags.

· Get organized. Label and date everything that's in a storage container.

· Let food cool completely before freezing. Placing warm food in the freezer can cause other items near it to thaw. Also, it takes forever to freeze warm food, which leads to a bacteria breeding ground.

· Ideally, thaw your food for a day or two in your refrigerator versus on the counter to prevent foodborne illnesses.

· The Food and Drug Administration (FDA) has a terrific guide to how long it is safe to freeze food items. Print it out and put it up on the fridge for easy reference.

· If you make a big dish with lots of servings and plan to freeze it, divide it into several containers. That way you can remove individual portions as needed.

> · I love freezing sauces in an ice cube tray. Once they're frozen, I transfer them to a silicone bag for easy storage. This allows you to serve individual portions—and consider it practice for making and storing baby food. (Trust me, ice cube trays will be your number-one kitchen item when you transition to solids.)

THINK ABOUT FEEDING

In the third trimester, you are probably taking labor and baby CPR classes and making decisions about how you want to feed your baby (breastfeeding, formula, or a combo). Even if you are dead set on nursing, things don't always go as planned—or you may change your mind—so you need a formula plan. This is even more important given the 2022 formula shortage, and while there have been massive strides to prevent a similar situation, you can never be too careful.

We are fortunate to have access to standardized formula with all the nutrients that a baby needs to thrive; beyond that, it's mostly a personal preference, so ask folks you trust about their experiences. I recommend choosing a formula that has received the Clean Label Project Purity Award, which means it's been independently tested to ensure that it is free from over four hundred contaminants and toxins. Of course, you can't stock up on anything this early, as your baby may have allergies or sensitivities that require them to have a specialty formula. Your pediatrician will guide you if that's the case. (Bear in mind that homemade infant formula won't meet your baby's essential nutritional needs and can even be dangerous to their growth and development. Homemade infant formula is not sterile, and it introduces many sources of bacterial contamination. You will have many opportunities for DIY motherhood; this is not one.)

If you plan to nurse and enroll in a lactation class, take your partner. When my husband tagged along, he learned so much that he was actually excited to wake up for some middle-of-the-night feedings and help (or at least commiserate) when an issue came up.

Finally, many hospitals and birthing centers have lactation consultants visit you after your baby's born, so check ahead to see if yours does.

FINAL CONSIDERATIONS

A few more items on the nesting to-do list. Spend a few moments considering the following:

- **Your placenta:** Some women choose to have their placenta encapsulated (meaning dehydrated, crushed into powder, and put into capsules) by a trusted professional, or they cook it up and eat it. The placenta is full of nutrients, and while the science is scarce, anecdotal evidence suggests it may assist with milk production and prevent postpartum depression. If you want your placenta encapsulated, hire the professional beforehand as they'll explain how to get it home safely. Most hospitals will require you to sign a form before they release the placenta, and you should bring a cooler with you.

- **Delayed umbilical cord clamping:** Until recently, most doctors cut the umbilical cord immediately after birth. Today, many hospitals delay cord clamping because research shows that even just an extra five minutes with the cord intact will increase hemoglobin levels in the baby and improve iron stores in the first several months of life. However, you may have to ask—and even insist—to have this done at your hospital, so be sure to discuss this with your provider before you give birth.

- **Delayed washing:** Nurses used to whisk a newborn away and return with them freshly washed and swaddled. While some hospitals still do this, it's not evidence-based or recommended anymore. Vernix caseosa—the white film that covers a baby after birth—protects the skin and is a rich source of bacteria that helps to build their microbiome. A recent study in the *Journal for Obstetrics, Gynecologic, and Neonatal Nursing* showed that waiting at least twenty-four hours before bathing supports breastfeeding too. Finally, baths cause temperature shifts, and remember that your baby just went from a balmy 98.6-degree environment to room temperature; no need to make them colder. Talk to your doctor about skipping the baby bath and simply wiping the newborn with a little warm water after twelve hours. There's just no reason for an instant bath.

FOODS TO INDUCE LABOR

You may feel *so* ready to have your baby, especially if you're past week forty, not sleeping well, feeling like you're carrying a small grizzly bear inside you, or are having contractions that turn out to be a false alarm. I wish I could say, "Eat this and, *voilà!* You'll be in labor." But I can't. There's no real evidence that any one food can bring on labor or make it smooth and easy. Unless you are induced, a baby comes when they're ready, so think of this as an exercise in having patience (something you'll soon need in spades).

All that said, let's talk about two foods:

· **Red raspberry leaf tea:** Women have been drinking this herbal infusion for centuries to bring on labor, and while there's little evidence that it can induce contractions, some research shows it may shorten the second stage of labor by an average of nine minutes. Red raspberry leaf tea is fragrant and tastes good—like a fruity black tea—so you may find it comforting to drink in the third trimester. You never know, it may help you in labor too, and there are no known contraindications.

· **Dates:** While I was pregnant with my daughter, Remi, I made weekly trips to my local favorite Middle Eastern bakery, Damascus Bakery in Brooklyn (a must-go-to when in Brooklyn; you'll thank me later). Once when I was checking out, the store owner grabbed a bag of fresh Medjool dates

and said, "You must have these; they are good for labor."
I trusted him and started snacking. Guess what? Remi's
delivery was *fast*. Now, whether that was because she was
my second or because of the dates, I will never know. But
science does suggest that there's something to be said for
dates, which contain fatty acids that help produce
prostaglandins, hormonelike substances that soften the
cervix. One study looked at a small sample of women who
consumed six dates a day for four weeks at the end of their
pregnancies, and they went into labor faster and dilated
more rapidly than the control group. Dates are also rich in
fiber, magnesium, potassium, and copper. Like other dried
fruits, they are high in sugar, so try to keep to two or three,
and for a snack, pair them with a protein (for example, a
handful of walnuts). If you have gestational diabetes, take a
pass or see how your body reacts to one (again, paired with a
protein).

Here are my top ways to enjoy dates:

· Stuffed with nut butter, tahini, or goat cheese

· Almond butter chocolate turtles: Stuff each date with
  roughly one teaspoon of almond butter and roll in melted
  chocolate (melt half a cup of dark chocolate with one
  tablespoon of coconut oil). Top with a little flaky sea salt and
  pop in the freezer to set, removing any excess chocolate that
  pools around the edges once frozen. To make them easier to
  chew, let them defrost before diving in.

· Add one or two dates to your smoothie

· Energy Bites (page 261)

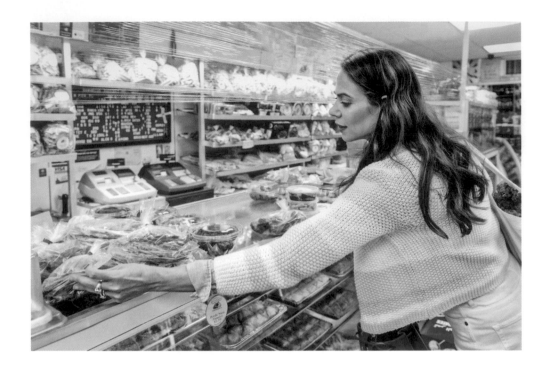

FOOD AND BEVERAGE FOR ACTIVE LABOR

When I was packing my hospital bag in preparation for my son's birth, food was the last thing on my mind. I just wanted everything to go smoothly and to get home as soon as possible. I didn't for a second think about snacks to get me through a potentially arduous labor, or for just waiting around for the show to start. I didn't even know what the hospital policies were around food.

I was thus completely blindsided when I was told I could eat *nothing* after I was induced with Pitocin. I quickly realized that water and Jell-O weren't going to cut it when my labor extended over twenty-four hours. Ask any person who's gone through it; active labor is incredibly demanding work physically and emotionally.

For this kind of intense workout, you need fuel. Unfortunately, when a woman gives birth in a hospital (as most American women do), she is often told not to eat or drink during labor to keep her stomach empty in case she needs emergency surgery with general anesthesia. (Many birthing centers are more flexible.) But is this no-food policy effective and necessary? The jury's still out on this one.

For now, if your hospital has this protocol in place, this is what I recommend. When you're still at home in early labor, aim for a light meal, if possible. This should be a food that you know you'll tolerate and digest well (this is not the time for fun surprises). Then, throughout labor, keep the snacks listed below on hand if your hospital will allow it. They'll provide quick energy and good hydration, so make, freeze, and pack what you can before your big day.

- **Dates:** Not only can they soften the cervix during labor, but their high sugar content provides an energy boost.

- **Honey sticks:** Delicious, easy to pack, and they recharge you fast.

- **Bone broth:** Nourishing and comforting, and the real bonus is that since it's a liquid, it is allowed at any hospital, even if they don't permit other food.

LIQUIDS FOR LABOR

Don't forget to pack your water bottle. Hydration is just as—if not more—important than eating during labor. While a lot of physicians rely on IV fluid (which is just saline water for electrolytes), drinking as much as you can after each contraction, both early on and into active labor, is a good rule of thumb. Some options:

- Coconut water
- Electrolyte packets mixed in water
- Watermelon water
- Popsicles: Refreshing and wonderful for an energy boost. Freeze coconut water (with berries or without), red raspberry leaf tea, and/or watermelon juice in ice cube trays, then pack in a cooler bag for the hospital—instant refreshment and better than ice chips from the hospital ice maker.

· Labor-Ade: There are many versions of this electrolyte-packed drink, but I love the one that follows. Freeze it in an ice cube tray, or pack a full bottle to bring to the hospital or birthing center.

INGREDIENTS

3 cups coconut water

1½ cups water

1½ tablespoons honey—local and raw is ideal,
   but use what you have

Juice of 2 lemons

Juice of 2 limes

½ teaspoon unrefined sea salt

Combine all the ingredients and enjoy.

SNACKS AFTER DELIVERY

You did it! And now you're *starving*. I scarfed down my bagel and lox spread as soon as it arrived in my hospital room, and you'd better believe I enjoyed it. Since not every woman has a full meal planned out in advance—and since no one should be forced to rely on hospital food for nourishment—toss a few snacks in your hospital bag or ask a friend or family member to bring them when they visit. (You can also eat these during early labor if you and your doctor feel comfortable.)

Consider how you like to eat after a workout. You just went through ten months of exhausting work for this moment, and now you can treat and replenish yourself. Try a combination of quick-acting carbohydrates and proteins, plus lots of liquids to rehydrate you (you just lost a lot of fluid, after all). Eat what feels good and satisfying, and don't hyperfocus on structure and timing. Listen to your body, and if you are hungry, eat! Your body needs it.

Here are some ideas:

· Energy Bites (page 261)

· Your favorite muffin (check out the Carrot Cake Muffins on page 206)

· Greek yogurt/yogurt parfait

· Banana or zucchini bread

· Bone broth (see page 247)

· Trail mix

· Granola bar (see page 203)

· Peanut butter and jelly sandwich

· High-protein smoothie

· Fresh fruit

· Turkey or beef jerky

A FINAL NOTE

After delivery, you may go through a dizzying range of emotions, from joy to what-the-heck-just-happened disorientation to shock that you're suddenly responsible for another human life. The sheer magnitude of becoming a mother doesn't start and stop in the moments and days after birth. Every single day of being a mom is different—some days are wonderful, some physically exhausting, some baffling (you smeared *what* on the carpet?!). The second you hear that first beautiful cry, you are the caretaker, cheerleader, disciplinarian, champion, hugger, and Mama Bear. It's all amazing, so snuggle that little baby of yours, because they're the best—and they're all yours. I am so happy for you!

SECTION FOUR: THE FOURTH TRIMESTER

Congratulations! You made it. But while a whole new life lies ahead, I want you first to take a moment, breathe deeply, and give yourself some love. You did something very difficult, you have a beautiful new baby, and you took care of yourself in the process.

While lots of women think things can only get easier after the flashy main event, they often don't—especially in those first few months. You're tired, overwhelmed, full of hormones and big emotions, starving, and exhausted. Oh, and there's a baby you have to take care of, nurture, love, and help grow. No pressure.

The icing on the cake, though, is the societal and internal pressure to "bounce back." I get the urge to push through—I have felt it firsthand—but this is the moment for emotional and physical healing. It's important to understand that you can't rush things, that you need to go at your own pace, and that you have to focus on what feels right for you and your baby—and nobody else.

This section covers the fourth trimester, the overlooked, underappreciated, and—as I said before—oftentimes toughest part of pregnancy and birth. As you learn about recovery, feeding, and becoming a mom, know that healthy nutrition can help you be a better mother and a happier, healthier person. Let's set you on a path of good eating habits that will hopefully last for years to come through all the wild, unexpected, and magnificent moments.

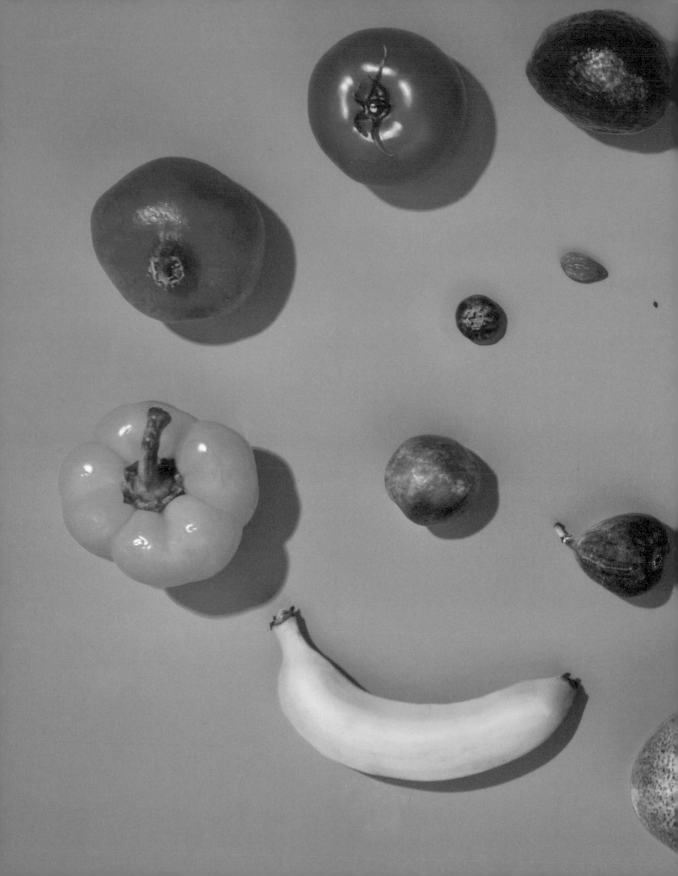

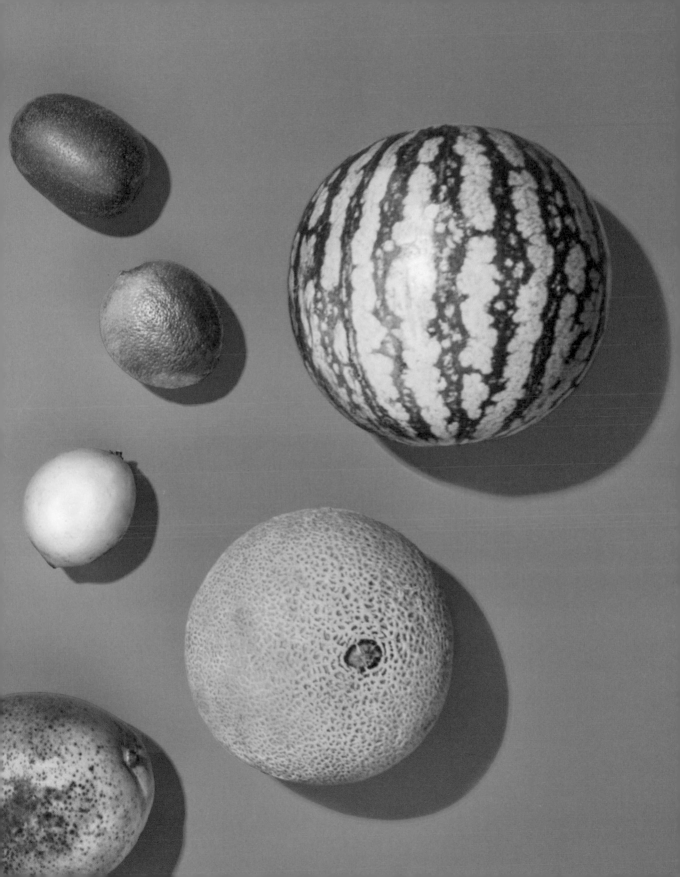

CHAPTER 9

FOODS FOR RECOVERY

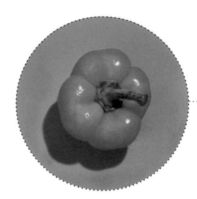

YOUR UTERUS IS THE
SIZE OF A PEPPER A FEW
DAYS AFTER GIVING
BIRTH.

Don't be surprised if everyone showers attention on your baby and hardly notices you. That's why you have to learn to take care of yourself from the start. The first step toward that essential self-care is to understand what's going on with your newly not-pregnant body and then to adjust your expectations accordingly. Even though recovery doesn't happen overnight, you will get there, and even though your body may feel different, you're just an improved version of the same old you.

WHAT RECOVERY LOOKS LIKE

Healing takes time. While there is no set timeline for postpartum recovery, and everyone has their own experience, below is a basic framework of what to expect after childbirth. It's not always pretty, and it may feel weird or gross at times, but again, your body has gone through a massive, life-changing event, and it needs time to adjust.

The first few days

- **Cramping:** You may experience cramping, which is due to the uterus shrinking back to its pre-pregnancy size.

- **Bleeding:** You will experience bleeding, and it may be heavy. This bleeding is called lochia, and it consists of blood, mucus, and uterine tissue. Do not be alarmed. Your body is letting go of everything that kept your baby safe and secure during pregnancy, and it's perfectly natural. Pads and giant mesh underwear will be your best friends after childbirth, so make sure to grab as many as you can on your way out of the hospital or birthing center. (If the bleeding gets heavier instead of lighter after the first few days, slow down a bit, as it could be a sign that your body needs more time to recover.)

- **Hormonal shifts:** From the moment you give birth, your progesterone and estrogen levels plummet, dropping as much as 1,000 percent in only a few days. You may find yourself suddenly depressed, moody, or anxious, all of which are normal unless they become severe. Later in this chapter, I'll describe how nutrition can help you cope and recover, as well as when you should seek outside assistance.

- **Breasts and milk production:** Your milk may come in—meaning you will produce more transitional breastmilk rather than colostrum (the antibody-rich yellowish substance you produce after birth)—typically a few days postpartum, and it may be accompanied by breast and nipple soreness or tenderness. If you had a C-section or an especially hard labor, it might take longer for you to produce milk. In the next chapter, I'll talk more about the foods that will benefit you while you're lactating.

- **Exhaustion:** Giving birth is a lot of work, and a C-section is major abdominal surgery. Regardless of how you delivered your baby, you will likely be exhausted. Please request support from family, friends, or anyone who will allow you to take the time you need to rest and recover.

- **Constipation and your first poop:** It may be hard to poop after childbirth because of pain medications, your new sleep schedule (or lack thereof), or dehydration. Contemplating your first poop may feel a bit scary, given you are sore in the vaginal and perineal areas, or—if you had a C-section—all over your abdomen. Treat constipation just as you did before you had the baby, with magnesium, hydration, fiber from green, leafy vegetables, chia seeds, ground flaxseed, and/or electrolytes. I also recommend the game-changing Squatty Potty. Some doctors may suggest stool softeners, which are fine, but avoid laxatives. You want your body to start to function on its own without the use of harsh medication.

- **Water retention:** If you received IV fluids at the hospital (which happens if you have an epidural, are given Pitocin to induce labor, or have a C-section), you may retain water after giving birth. I was incredibly swollen after leaving the hospital—way more than when I arrived. I could barely get shoes on for the first visit with our pediatrician. This swelling should go away in a few days, or up to a week, but if it doesn't, reach out to your doctor.

Weeks one to two

- **Bleeding:** Your bleeding and discharge should taper off by the end of week two, moving from a bright red to a brownish red to light pink (just like a period). Your discharge may even be yellow. That's okay.

- **Soreness:** If you had a vaginal delivery, you may still notice soreness or swelling down there. Your vagina just had the biggest workout of its life, so this is to be expected. If you had a C-section, your stitches may hurt quite a lot, but if the pain becomes severe, talk to your doctor.

Months one to three

- **Soreness:** If you had a vaginal delivery, your perineum may still feel sore. If you had a C-section, the pain from your incision will have decreased, but you may still ache. Give it time. The pain will pass.

- **Ovulation:** Around day forty-five, most women have their first postpartum ovulation, though you may not have a period, especially if you're breastfeeding. Be sure to have a plan for contraception if you're sexually active and don't want to get pregnant again. The myth that you can't get pregnant while breastfeeding is, in fact, a myth.

- **Diastasis recti:** While many women's abdominal muscles move back to their pre-pregnancy positions by six weeks, about 60 percent of women still have diastasis recti, which is abdominal separation resulting in a pooch. Ten percent of women still experience this a year postpartum. Certain exercises can help repair diastasis recti. Also, ask your provider for a referral to see a postpartum physical therapist—they are angels with the sole goal of alleviating these kinds of conditions.

Months three and on

- **Hair loss:** Most women have glorious pregnancy hair because of the rise in estrogen, but by six months postpartum, it begins to shed as hormone levels drop. Postpartum hair loss is common, but luckily it's usually not permanent. I hope that's a relief because, with everything else going on in your life, the last thing you need is to mourn those vibrant, thick tresses. There's not a magic pill you can take to grow back that hair, but a diet rich in protein, fatty acids, and vitamins A, C, D, E, and B, plus biotin, iron, zinc, and copper can help. Continue to take your prenatal and eat plenty of meat, eggs, fish, and colorful fruits and vegetables. In short, do what you've been doing, and if you keep losing hair past month six and it's not back to prenatal levels, have your thyroid tested, as hypothyroidism (which can be triggered by pregnancy) can lead to hair loss.

YOUR SIX-WEEK APPOINTMENT

Most women are eager for their six-week postpartum appointment, partly because you'll usually get the okay to exercise again (*gently* if you had a C-section). In addition to completing a postpartum depression questionnaire, this is the time to tell your provider about any issues that are weighing on you: soreness, how your C-section or episiotomy incision is healing, when it's physically okay to have sex, whether you'd like a referral for postpartum physical therapy, etc.

Ask for updated labs too. You want to get a sense of your levels of vitamins B_{12} and D and iron, in particular, as well as reassess your blood sugar levels and blood pressure (if that was a concern during pregnancy). Request blood work to monitor your hormone levels and a full thyroid panel, too, since imbalances can cause depression and mood swings. You don't want to get a prescription for an antidepressant when your thyroid is the issue, and I have seen that happen. The National Institutes of Health (NIH) reports that 5 percent of postpartum women experience thyroiditis, which is an inflamed thyroid that leads to dysfunction. That's a huge problem that next to no one talks about, but luckily it's easily treatable—*if* it is spotted and diagnosed correctly.

NUTRITION FOR RECOVERY

During the fourth trimester, your nutrient needs are actually higher than they were when you were pregnant. It sounds counterintuitive, but think about it. First, your body just went through a major event, and you need proper nutrition to heal from the physical exertion of labor. Your body also carried a baby for almost ten months, and a lot of the nutrition you took in went to them, depleting your stores. Last, if you are nursing, your body needs a big boost to feed and nourish your little one. (I'll talk about that more in the next chapter.)

The term for "being behind where you should be" after birth is *postnatal depletion*. While postnatal depletion refers to the general sense of exhaustion, fatigue, insufficiency ("I'm not doing enough"), brain fog, and distractedness that many postpartum women feel, its roots lie in poor nutrition. Not only did you give your main stores of vitamins and minerals to your baby in the womb (in particular, iron, zinc, calcium, vitamin B_{12}, vitamin B_9, iodine, selenium, docosahexaenoic acid [DHA], and certain amino acids from proteins), but you may not be getting the nutrition you need. Once you give birth, you may find yourself so distracted by nursing, soothing baby's crying, and swaddling that you ignore your own nutritional needs, eating whatever casserole your aunt or neighbor made or snacking on chips and other processed foods. A postpartum woman needs about 500 more calories a day than she did before she was pregnant, which is about two hundred more than when she was pregnant. And women who are exclusively breastfeeding need an extra 670 calories a day.

To make sure you're getting your body what it needs to heal, focus on the following nutrients and food categories. I encourage you to consult the chart on page 16 for a list of which foods contain which nutrients:

- **Protein:** Replenish and repair with protein, and put it on repeat. Pay special attention to the amino acid glycine and the protein collagen, which together repair the tissue that shifted around or broke down during pregnancy and childbirth.

- **Fats:** Healthy fats nourish and fuel your metabolism. They also build and enrich your milk supply and support the absorption of nutrients, especially fat-soluble vitamins. They play a role in hormone production and lubricate your intestines, keeping you regular.

- **Hydration:** You lost a lot of electrolytes during labor, and if you're breastfeeding, your chances of becoming dehydrated are high. If you're nursing, add more electrolytes because you're providing so much in your milk. Aim for room temperature or warm liquids, as they are much easier on your system after delivery than cold beverages.

- **Iron:** Many women go into pregnancy iron deficient, then deplete any additional iron stores. You also lose a lot of blood in birth, so be sure you're getting enough iron. Postpartum anemia is a real risk. See page 42 for more on iron-rich foods and how to boost iron stores.

- **Vitamin C:** Vitamin C strengthens your immune system and bolsters collagen production, which you'll need as your tissues repair themselves. Aim for two servings of vitamin C–rich foods a day.

- **Vitamin B$_{12}$:** B vitamins are central to energy level and mental health, and mothers are frequently deficient. Years after my second pregnancy, I can still become low in iron and B$_{12}$ if I don't keep an eye on it.

- **DHA:** DHA is vital for repairing the brain and nervous system, and a sleep-deprived new mom needs to stay sharp. Low levels are linked to cognitive decline, depression, and your body's inability to handle stress.

- **Choline:** Choline can also reduce the risk of postpartum anxiety and depression.

- **Iodine:** Iodine needs are highest in postpartum women who are nursing, particularly for thyroid health, which needs some TLC after delivery. You can find it in foods like seaweed, eggs, and seafood and dairy such as yogurt, cheese, and kefir.

- **Vitamin D:** Recommended levels of vitamin D for nursing moms are even higher than those in pregnancy. Continue taking your vitamin D_3 supplement, and at your postpartum visit, ask to get your levels retested so you know if you need to tweak the dosage. Or better yet, get outside as much as you can. Sunshine is nature's vitamin D!

- **Probiotics:** These good bacteria are your postpartum buddies. If you weren't taking a probiotic supplement during pregnancy, consider taking one now, especially if you were put on antibiotics during or right after labor or your baby was born via C-section. You should also seek out probiotic-rich food sources like fermented vegetables, yogurt, miso, and kefir. As discussed on page 144, there is a ton of research dedicated to the gut microbiome in relation to chronic immune-related conditions in kids (like eczema and allergies). Building up the microbiome is also particularly crucial in the first one to two months of breastfeeding.

WARMING FOODS FOR COMFORT AND NUTRITION

Across all cultures, warming foods are cherished in the postpartum space because they provide comfort and are grounding. They're soothing, easy to digest, and nutrient-dense, and the ones listed below are high in fat and protein to support your milk supply, replenish your blood, and repair tissue.

- **Bone broth:** Bone Broth (page 247) provides collagen and minerals, like zinc, iron, and selenium, as well as hydration. You can make it or easily purchase it online or in the store. Check out organic and grass-fed beef broths for a big dose of iron, or if you don't eat meat, go for a veggie-based version. Sip bone broth on its own like tea or use it as a base for soups, stews, and rice dishes—simply replace any water or liquid that is called for in the recipe with broth.

- **Protein-rich soups and stews:** In the recipe section (see page 187), I've included several delicious and satisfying soups and stews that you can make ahead and freeze. They are easy to reheat and eat, and you can even drink them out of a mug if sitting down to a meal feels out of reach. For plant-based eaters, you can rely on beans and lentils in your stews and meals to give you that same hearty, nourishing experience.

WHAT ABOUT MY SUPPLEMENTS?

Again, keep taking your prenatals. Your baby took from your vitamin stores for almost ten months, so you need to build them back up. If you took supplemental vitamin D, DHA, or probiotics (especially if you were put on antibiotics following delivery or had an infection), don't skip those either. If you're not nursing, continue taking prenatals for at least six months postpartum, and if you are nursing, take them for six months *after* you wean.

FOOD AND MOOD

More than anything else I tell you, remember this: if you are experiencing severe depression, anxiety, fatigue, brain fog, or any other issues that are impacting your ability to function, seek help from a professional. The National Institute of Mental Health (NIMH) estimates that 15 percent of new moms experience postpartum depression. My guess is that this number, which is already extraordinarily high, is underreported. The good news is that, with the right treatments and support, you can feel better.

That said, one of the causes of postpartum depression (PPD) is the severe nutritional deficiencies many new moms experience. One study even laid out the case that eating a wide and sufficient variety of vegetables, fruits, legumes, seafood, milk and dairy products, and olive oil can reduce PPD by as much as 50 percent. The research suggests that women who experience PPD may be low in the following:

· B vitamins (B_6, B_{12}, and folate)

· Magnesium

· Vitamin D

· DHA

· Vitamin C

· Zinc

· Selenium

· Iron

Take care of yourself. There is no timeline for recovery, nor is there a one-size-fits-all model for what recovery looks like. Try to get support, rest, adjust your expectations, learn to go with the flow, meet other new parents, move your body (slowly at first), and eat nutrient-dense foods. You are the best mom you can be, and you should be proud of that.

CHAPTER 10

NUTRITION FOR NURSING

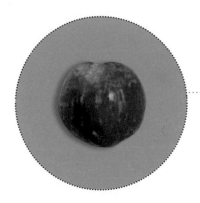

YOUR UTERUS IS THE
SIZE OF A PLUM, ITS
PRE-PREGNANCY SIZE,
AROUND SIX WEEKS
AFTER GIVING BIRTH.

All right, mama, I will preface this entire chapter with this: nursing is hard. While it can be rewarding and fulfilling, it can also feel challenging, painful, exhausting, and endless, and it may not work out. That's okay. There are a million personal and societal pressures surrounding nursing—not to mention a zillion opinions about what's best for you and your baby—which can lead to feeling overwhelmed and stressed. Having a bad nursing day can set the tone for how you feel emotionally, especially if you were dead set on doing it "perfectly." Be kind to yourself. The process is different for every mother. There is no one right way to feed your child.

BREASTFEEDING RECOMMENDATIONS

I'll be blunt: if you're on the fence, I highly recommend trying to breastfeed. In the first few days after birth, breastfeeding helps build your baby's immune system and microbiome by supplying them with antibodies and beneficial bacteria. It also lowers your risk of breast cancer, hypertension, and diabetes. But if you can't breastfeed for whatever reason, know that babies also build up their microbiome through skin-to-skin contact by passing through the vaginal canal and with the vernix caseosa. The pressure we put on new mothers is intense, and it is *so* not worth it to torture yourself. Fed is best.

My goal is to set you up for breastfeeding from a nutritional, educational, and emotional standpoint, so let's start with the guidelines from the American Academy of Pediatrics (AAP): You should try to breastfeed from birth up to two years or beyond. Now, for many of you that is completely unrealistic. If you've gone back to work and have little time to pump; if you have other children running around who need you; or if you are tired or not producing enough, nursing or pumping may be such a strain that it's time to supplement with formula or give up entirely. I aimed to nurse for three months, then six months, then more, until it just didn't feel right anymore for me *or* my children. No judgment!

My main suggestion is to seek support. Nursing is as much technique as it is art. Many hospitals provide free consultations with lactation consultants, and you should absolutely, positively take them up on it, even if nursing is going well for you. Research in advance if your hospital or birthing center provides these services, and if they don't, reach out to a lactation consultant or counselor to schedule a postpartum visit. If seeing a lactation consultant is not an option for you, take a breastfeeding class. If that's not an option, find a new mom friend who is nursing, and sit with them while they nurse (if they are comfortable with that). You will learn a lot and have plenty to talk (and complain) about. If that feels odd or if you don't have nursing friends, the La Leche League, which aims to support breastfeeding, has branches in over eighty countries, offers a wealth of information online, and provides online and in-person support groups, no matter how young or old your child is.

WHAT'S IN BREAST MILK?

I'm obsessed with ingredients, and breast milk is no exception. If you're feeding it to your baby, you should know what's in it, right? One of the fascinating things about breast milk is that it completely changes based on what you eat, the time of day, and your baby's needs. For example, if your baby gets sick, your milk will soon contain more antibodies to help them get better.

Milk is composed of protein, lactose, fat (which provides a baby 50 percent of their energy needs), and the minerals calcium, phosphorus, magnesium, potassium, sodium, and chloride. Starting on day one of your baby's life, your milk goes through several stages:

- **Colostrum:** This thick (sometimes chunky) yellow or orangish liquid appears soon after birth and typically up to five days after; some women will have noticed it leaking weeks ahead of childbirth. It's full of protein, low in lactose, and rich in antibodies. It also has a laxative effect that helps your baby take their first poop.

- **Transitional milk (days five to fourteen):** This milk is high in lactose, sugars, enzymes, and fat, all of which help your baby put on weight and poop a lot.

- **Mature milk (day fourteen and on):** This is lower in protein than colostrum but higher in fat and carbohydrates. It also contains a lot of water to keep your baby hydrated and tends to have a sweeter taste than colostrum or transitional milk.

What does breast milk taste like to your baby? It's sweet and fatty and slightly flavored by the foods you eat. Formula always tastes the same unless you switch brands.

FOODS FOR NURSING

Heads up, mamas. When you are nursing round-the-clock, you will be starving. It's a hunger you have never experienced before, and it will likely shock you. I felt this way, as has every single new mom I work with. What can you eat to satisfy your cravings, meet your nutritional needs, and ensure your milk is high quality?

Let's home in on that last one, because is there even such a thing as high-quality milk? This is something a lot of moms wonder and worry about, causing the mom guilt to go from zero to sixty in no time. Your breast milk is constantly evolving, so what you eat in a single day or meal will never make or break your quality or supply. If you eat not-so-healthy one day, it doesn't mean your baby is going to suffer, as long as you find your way back to good nutrition sooner or later. Food should be about nourishment and enjoyment, so don't hyperfocus on the macronutrients.

The recipes in part two will support you and your milk supply, but the first and most critical thing to remember is that you have to eat enough. Many nursing moms are just not consuming enough food for a variety of reasons, including stress, lack of time, or the need or pressure to "get their bodies back." Coupled with the fact that your nutritional needs are much higher than in pregnancy, you need to fuel yourself first.

Eat more of everything: fats, proteins, complex carbohydrates, fruits, and veggies. Because breast milk is primarily composed of fat, lean toward foods like avocados, nuts, seeds, healthy oils (olive, coconut, avocado), meat, fish, and full-fat dairy. An equally key consideration is hydration. Aim to get in eight ounces of water during each nursing session, with your overall consumption of ninety to one hundred ounces a day. Water alone will not be enough to satisfy your needs when it comes to sodium, potassium, and magnesium, so include a drink rich with electrolytes at least once a day. I drank at least sixteen ounces of coconut water daily, but you can also try watermelon water and electrolyte mixes. Proper hydration is more than just water.

While eating a wide variety of healthy foods, and a lot of it, should be enough to support your nursing journey, there are certain lactogenic foods that build up your milk supply: oats, flaxseed, barley, brewer's yeast, chia seeds, beans, lentils, nuts, and seeds. When I was nursing, I ate oats with flaxseed and chia seeds every day (hello energy bites, bars, cookies, baked oatmeal); you can simply cook up a bowl of oatmeal with a sprinkling of flaxseed and nuts for the same results. Like many women, I felt these lactogenic foods helped maintain my supply, but there isn't much data to back that feeling up. Perhaps eating these kinds of supportive, nutrient-filled meals feels proactive, helpful, and loving, and those good feelings stimulate the hormones prolactin and oxytocin, which lets down our milk. Either way, there's no downside to eating these healthy and nourishing foods, so go for it.

SUPPLEMENTS FOR BREASTFEEDING

Galactagogues (including the herbs fenugreek, milk thistle, and nettle) are foods that have a reputation for improving your milk supply, although, as with the foods for nursing that I went over above, there isn't much hard science to prove they work. There aren't side effects associated with drinking infusions or taking supplements of these herbs, and many women swear by them, so feel free to try them if you need a boost to your milk supply.

Another option is prescription drugs with long names, including metoclopramide, domperidone, chlorpromazine, and sulpiride, but they have side effects, including dry mouth, GI upset, hypertension, and exhaustion. Before asking for a prescription, I recommend shifting your diet to improve your milk supply and trying more skin-to-skin contact before and while breastfeeding. Skin-to-skin may increase levels of prolactin and oxytocin in your body, which release your milk.

Regular pumping also increases supply and letdown. If you're pumping while away from your baby, look at a photo of them while you're hooked up. Seeing their sweet little face can get those happy hormones up and running, and you'll notice your milk comes in faster.

FOODS TO AVOID DURING NURSING

Good news: there are no foods you have to avoid when you're breastfeeding. Store-bought salads, soft cheeses, and cold cuts . . . bring them on. Eat whatever nutritious foods you like, whenever you like, unless you notice an obvious reaction in your baby. If you have a family history of allergies or think your baby might be allergic to a certain food or type of food (common allergens are dairy, eggs, nuts, seafood, wheat, and soy), try cutting it out for a week and notice any changes.

You may have heard that eating certain foods—typically cruciferous veggies like broccoli, cauliflower, cabbage, kale, and Brussels sprouts—will make your baby gassy. The answer is maybe. Breastmilk is made from what passes into the blood, not the GI tract, so if a mother gets gas from certain foods, her child won't necessarily have the same reaction. Most babies are also just gassy little creatures, so again, pay attention to your baby's patterns, or lack of them. If your baby spits up excessively or fusses a lot after you eat a particular food, take note. Skip it for a while and see if things improve. Just bear in mind that at around one month of age, a lot of babies develop acid reflux because their digestive systems change, and this has little to do with your diet.

WHAT ABOUT CAFFEINE AND ALCOHOL?

After nine-plus months of being careful about caffeine, and now sleep-deprived and hazy, you're wondering if that cup (or three) of coffee is okay. According to research, caffeine is safe while breastfeeding, and one study shows that caffeine consumption by nursing mothers has no effect on a baby's sleep at three months of age. Some babies are extra sensitive, so as with foods, watch their responses and sleep patterns after you consume it.

I recommend sticking to one regular—not large—cup of organic coffee per day (since conventionally grown beans are high in pesticides and mycotoxins) and/or working in other caffeinated beverages, like green or black tea. Even though coffee is safe for your milk, drinking two or more cups can leave you jittery and anxious and make your physiological highs higher and your lows lower, so that when you're down, you crave more to get you back up. Finally, when you drink coffee, you often forget to drink water, and dehydration can impact milk levels—so if you are going for the joe, make sure to match it cup for cup with water or another hydrating beverage.

Now . . . drumroll . . . let's chat about alcohol. This is probably the single most misunderstood, judged, and guilt-inducing topic while nursing. Once, I had a glass of wine at a restaurant with my newborn in my arms, and I got plenty of funny looks from total strangers. Let's get the facts straight. According to research, a nursing baby is exposed to 5 to 6 percent of what the mother drinks and metabolizes. That's a bit confusing, so I'll sum it up: science says that a dose of that size is not clinically relevant. Still, drinking does affect a mother's let-down reflex, so she may produce less milk after drinking.

If a nursing mom drinks a few glasses of wine, she may feel she has to get rid of the milk. This is known as pumping and dumping. The rule of thumb is that for every standard-sized drink, it takes two hours for the alcohol to leave your body. For example, if you have two drinks, four hours later none will show up in your blood or milk. You get the math. You can certainly choose to express or pump after drinking if it works with your pumping schedule or if you're experiencing physical discomfort, and you may want to dispose of that breastmilk if it falls into the two-hour window. But you don't have to. Waiting until the alcohol has left your system, then nursing, works just as well.

TESTING BREAST MILK

If you are worried about what's in your breast milk—or just curious—some companies (see the resources on page 276) will test for its nutritional concentration as well as toxins like arsenic, lead, and other heavy metals. There is ample evidence that certain toxins can pass through a mother's body into her milk, so if you're worried about any kind of exposure or contamination, check out one of these places.

OPTIONS BEYOND BREASTFEEDING

Let me say this again, and this time louder: fed is best! If you are having trouble breastfeeding, can't produce sufficient milk for your baby, are tired of nursing, don't think it's right for you or your baby, or won't do it for reasons that are nobody's business but yours, you have a few options. Breastfeeding is not the right answer for every baby, mother, and situation, nor is it essential for a happy, healthy child.

Instead of breastfeeding, you can opt for the following:

- **Formula:** It's been amazing to see this space boom in the past few years, and there are many new(ish) formulas on the market. Find one that works for you and your baby and that you feel good about. See chapter 8 for more information on choosing the right formula.

- **Donor milk:** For any number of reasons (infant loss, excess milk production, etc.), some mothers donate to milk banks, and that milk is available to babies who are otherwise unable to breastfeed. Donated milk is tested for bacteria and diseases, pasteurized, and analyzed for its nutritional content, then donated to hospitals or families in need. In the resources section (see page 276) I've provided a link to milk banks across the US, where you can donate or apply to receive milk, if needed. Bear in mind there is a large demand for donor milk, so if you try for it, it's not guaranteed you will receive it.

WEIGHT LOSS

Postpartum weight loss is a brutal subject full of pressure and shame, and it's one of the most common topics I am asked about.

Here's what I tell my clients: be patient with yourself. For *at least* the first three months, don't even think about trying to lose weight, as your body needs to heal and recover. Those first few months are a blur, and your schedule will revolve around your baby. If you need to eat at 3:00 a.m., so be it. Once you and your baby get into a groove (and that will ebb and flow), then you can start to think about your eating structure. Or maybe not.

I know strong, healthy women who've been asked, "When's your baby due?" six months postpartum. Often, a mama's midsection and other parts of her body look different after birth due to diastasis recti, a change in exercise routines, or fluctuating hormones. Most women will lose about ten pounds immediately after birth (from the weight of the baby, amniotic fluid, and shrinking uterus), and about 50 percent of breastfeeding women lose their baby weight relatively quickly. Others don't. No matter who you are or what you weighed pre-pregnancy, your body is going to look different now, and you will carry more weight in certain areas. Nursing, going back to work, getting up in the middle of the night when your baby cries, the cost of diapers and formula, and the fact that your life is wildly different than it used to be are stressful. When your body is stressed, cortisol levels rise, making weight loss even tougher.

Again, your body not only needs to heal, but it also needs fuel, especially if you're nursing. So instead of restricting calories, let's talk about ways to establish a healthy and sustainable eating groove. A good meal routine is one that your whole family can follow, including your baby once they start eating regular meals, and one that will offer supportive lifelong eating habits for everyone.

CREATING A GREAT MEAL ROUTINE

As a new mom, it is sooooo hard to find structure. Your baby eats every few hours (and sometimes more than that), so you might lose track of whether it's 6 a.m. or time for lunch. Even if you've gotten a handle on taking in key nutrients, enough water, and all your supplements, you still may feel out of control. I see this *all the time* with my clients, and I have felt it myself.

I'll try to keep it simple. You can gain control back by planning ahead, doing some minor prep work, and being consistent with certain habits. What follows are my tips to keep things straightforward so you can devote your energy to loving on your new baby and taking time for self-care rather than standing over the stove.

- **Rely on make-ahead breakfasts:** Go for frittatas, eggs baked in muffin tins, baked oatmeal, overnight oats, chia seed puddings, and smoothies that you make ahead of time, pour into a container or glasses in individual servings, and put in the freezer. Mornings with a little one can be chaos, so planning sets the stage for a more carefree day.

- **Simplify your snacks:** Hit repeat and eat the same snacks over and over again. You crave what you eat, and snacks are no exception. Aim for a combination of DIY and on-the-go snacks. For a few weeks, you might rotate an apple and nut butter, avocado toast, yogurt with nuts, or a piece of Tahini Banana Bread (page 209) with butter.

- **Work one-handed:** Realize that for the foreseeable future, one of your hands will often be occupied. Think about eating one-handed snacks that are healthy and contain protein and fat—for example, a seed granola bar (see page 203), healthy muffin (see page 206), smoothie (see page 191; sip with a glass or silicone straw), Energy Bites (page 261), meatballs (see page 251), frittata (see page 193), or toast with nut butter, avocado, or hummus.

- **Stock your freezer:** Keep meats, fish, veggies, and fruits all stocked up so you can toss together easy meals based on what you have on hand.

- **Practice mindful eating:** If you find yourself constantly reaching for food, take a beat and tune in to your hunger cues. Try to figure out why you are eating. Remember HALT (hungry, anxious, lonely, or tired), and if you're not eating out of hunger, reach for water or tea first. If you are eating all day long, you're not letting yourself get hungry, so your body starts to expect never-ending snacks.

- **Double up on recipes:** When you do cook, make more than you need and freeze the leftovers in individually sized portions.

- **Cut corners:** Purchase pre-chopped veggies (even basics like garlic and onions); freeze sauces (like pesto—see page 229) in individual ice cube tray servings: batch cook things like rice and beans for the week or purchase organic heat-and-eat grains (heat them up in a microwave-safe dish, not whatever container they come in).

- **Make time for dinner with your partner:** It won't be every night, and you may have to plan weeks in advance, but eating together will help reconnect you and your partner. While I was pregnant, a friend advised that my husband and I pick a weekly date night once the baby was born. We kept to it, and I'm so glad we did. If this is your first kid, you'll be surprised at how impossible it can feel to have time together if you don't make a real point of it.

Can't stand the thought of planning *anything*? I'll make it easy for you. The chart that follows has a week of meal ideas to choose from. You don't need to follow this to a T; simply make as many as you like or as few. Double up on whatever strikes your fancy and save the rest for later. Most of all, enjoy.

	MONDAY	TUESDAY	WEDNESDAY
BREAKFAST	Apple and Pear Baked Oatmeal (page 266) topped with nut butter, tahini, or full-fat yogurt and Blueberry and Date Chia Jam (page 198)	Slice of Roasted Red Pepper and Asparagus Frittata (page 193), plus optional fresh fruit or sliced avocado	Chia pudding (see page 104), plus optional add-ins: nuts, shredded unsweetened coconut, and fruit
SNACK	Hummus and crackers	Banana with nut butter	Slice of Roasted Red Pepper and Asparagus Frittata (page 193) or hard-boiled eggs and fresh fruit
LUNCH	Leftover Breaded Chicken Cutlets (page 215) over greens and avocado or paired with Pickle-y Slaw	Leftover Citrusy Beet and Barley Salad (page 257)	Leftover Ginger Veggie Fried Rice (page 211)
SNACK	Yogurt parfait (plain full-fat yogurt with hempseed hearts, pumpkin seeds, sliced fruit, and a drizzle of honey or maple syrup)	Apple and Pear Baked Oatmeal (page 266) topped with full-fat yogurt	Energy Bites (page 261)
DINNER	Citrusy Beet and Barley Salad (page 257)	Ginger Veggie Fried Rice (page 211)	Classic Meatballs (page 251) over pasta or zucchini noodles, with roasted veggies of choice
NIGHT SNACK	· Energy Bites (page 261) · Chocolate Freezer Fudge Bites (page 267) · Avocado Chocolate Mousse (page 269) · Ice pop (see pages 271–273) · Slice of Tahini Banana Bread (page 209) · Yogurt with walnuts and a drizzle of honey		

THURSDAY	FRIDAY	SATURDAY	SUNDAY
Avocado toast topped with eggs and seasoning	Savory cottage cheese toast (full-fat cottage cheese over toast, topped with cucumbers, cherry tomatoes, and seasoning)	Green Smoothie (page 191) paired with a piece of Tahini Banana Bread (page 209) or a Carrot Cake Muffin (page 206)	Spinach Waffles (page 197) topped with nut butter, Cinnamon Honey Butter (page 198), or Blueberry and Date Chia Jam (page 198)
Chia pudding (see page 104)	Seaweed snacks and hummus	Homemade Granola Bar (page 203), plus optional fruit or nut butter/tahini	Cheddar cheese and sliced apple
Leftover Classic Meatballs (page 251) served over pasta, zucchini noodles, or a salad	Salmon Poke-Inspired Bowl (page 245) using leftover Sheet Pan Miso Salmon and Bok Choy (page 235)	Leftover Chicken Thighs with Roasted Carrots, Onions, and Chickpeas (page 239) with Crispy Baked Sweet Potato Fries (page 233)	Avocado/egg salad (see page 112) over a bed of greens or toast)
Carrot Cake Muffin (page 206) or a piece of Tahini Banana Bread (page 209) topped with ghee, grass-fed butter, or nut butter	PB&J Lactogenic Smoothie (page 263)	Savory cottage cheese (full-fat cottage cheese combined with cucumbers, cherry tomatoes, and everything bagel seasoning)	Leftover Crispy Baked Sweet Potato Fries (page 233) with tahini
Sheet Pan Miso Salmon and Bok Choy (page 235) with cooked rice	Chicken Thighs with Roasted Carrots, Onions, and Chickpeas (page 239)	Beef stew (see page 253) with roasted veggie of choice or a side salad	Breaded Chicken Cutlets with Pickle-y Slaw (page 215)

BEYOND THE FOURTH TRIMESTER

Well, that was quick. Time flies when you're having fun, right? I'm proud of you, but, more important, *you* should be proud of yourself. No matter how robust your support system, pregnancy and childbirth still fall squarely on one person's shoulders: yours. And that's a lot.

I hope this book has not only helped you through these past four trimesters but has set you on a path to a successful future. I'm so honored to have played a small part in it. Thank you for trusting me. Hopefully, what you've learned will translate into lifelong lessons, for you, for your baby, and for your growing family. Even though, going forward, you might not have to worry about some of what we've discussed, many of these topics will be applicable as your little one grows into a healthy toddler and beyond.

Congratulations, mama!

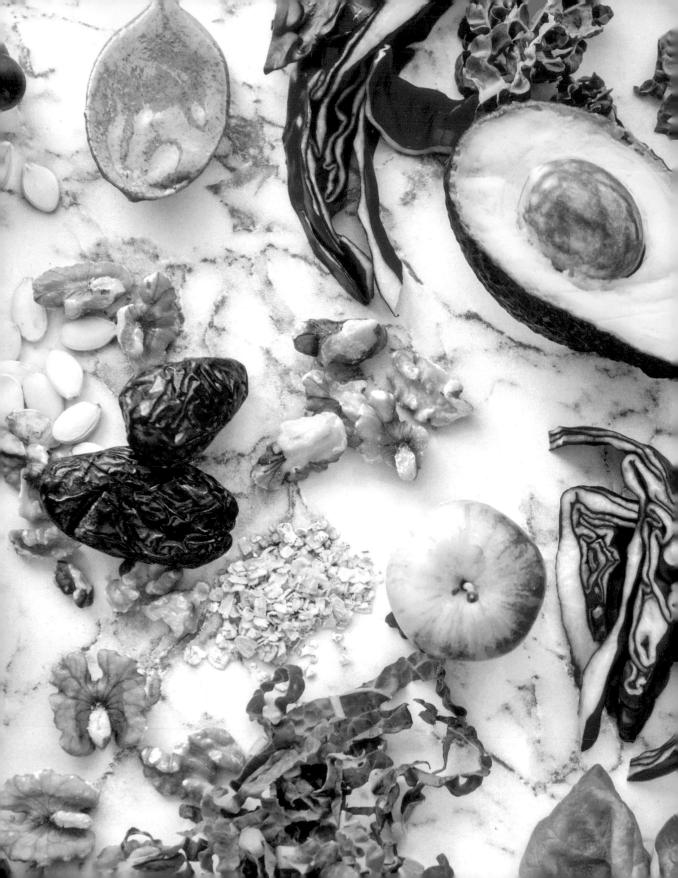

PART TWO

RECIPES

First and foremost, I wanted these recipes to be easy to make, easy to store, and easy to eat. They are crafted to satisfy as diverse a range of tastes and cravings as possible, and they're filled with nutrients that will achieve everything you've been striving for. Now, some are quick to make, and some require a bit more time and attention, but I promise all of them are worth the effort.

These are not just pregnancy meals, either. You can eat them while you're trying for a baby or when you're a grandmother, and everything in between. I've tried to be thoughtful about designing recipes that you can take with you well beyond the fourth trimester. Also, while many are free of the most common allergens, even the ones that aren't can be easily adapted.

As I've said a thousand times and truly believe, just do your best. If you need to cut corners, go for it. If the thought of doing a ton of prep makes you exhausted, then find some organic pre-chopped veggies, wash them well, and go to town. This is all about doing what's right for you and your family.

Recipes include the following:

· **Breakfasts:** Nutritious and delicious meals will inspire you and jump-start your day.

· **Baked goods:** I leaned heavily into these during and after pregnancy. They're not carb-filled bricks, though; quite the opposite! These treats are brimming with nutrients to fill you up and nurture you and baby. Make them ahead of time and freeze or eat as a meal or a rewarding snack.

· **Comfort foods:** These are healthified versions of your favorites (beef and broccoli, breaded chicken cutlets, ginger fried rice).

· **Veggies:** You need them, but sometimes they're the last thing you want. So this section includes options that make it easier to do the thing you're going to be saying for the next eighteen years: *Eat your veggies!*

· **Sheet pans and bowls:** Sheet pan meals are a delicious lifesaver, easy to make, and even easier to clean up.

· **Make-ahead meals:** These recipes include beef stew, lentil root veggie stew, meatballs, and lasagna. They are designed to live in the freezer for a while and taste just as fresh as if you had cooked them on the spot, while also being deeply fortifying and satisfying.

· **Lactogenic foods:** These are for the nursing mamas out there to boost your milk supply. Think energy bites, cookies, baked oatmeal; all are delicious, nurturing, and a piece of cake to make.

· **Sweets:** I had a sweet tooth in my pregnancies and had to include this section. These recipes will satisfy that sugar craving with zero guilt and without sacrificing flavor.

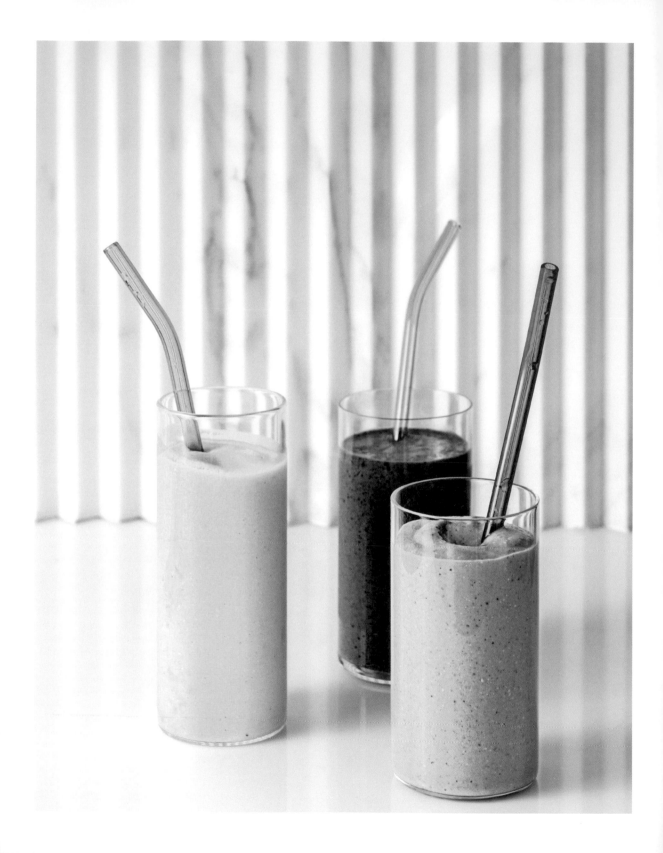

BREAKFASTS

Smoothies

PREP TIME: 10 MINUTES

On those days when you're feeling a little queasy, and a full meal isn't appealing, a smoothie is your solution. These pack a nutritional punch, are hydrating, and taste great. Putting a little something in your stomach can relieve the nausea, so try one in the morning to kick off the day or in the afternoon as a pick-me-up. Use fresh or frozen fruit except where specified. Simply combine all the ingredients in a high-speed blender, blend, and go. Add a scoop of collagen peptides or protein powder to make it even more filling.

Each of the recipes below makes one large (16-ounce) smoothie or two small (8-ounce) smoothies. If you have extra, try freezing it in ice-pop molds.

GREEN SMOOTHIE

Get your greens in with zero cooking. Especially if leafy greens aren't feeling appealing, this is a tasty way to consume them.

1/2 ripe avocado
1 kiwi, peeled
1/2 ripe banana
1/2 cup frozen mango chunks
1 cup packed baby spinach
2 tablespoons hempseed hearts

RECIPE CONTINUES

1 cup unsweetened almond milk or milk of choice

6 to 8 fresh basil leaves (optional)

BLUE SMOOTHIE

With plenty of vitamin C, folate, potassium, and fiber, blueberries are a pregnant person's friend (it helps that they're sweet and juicy too). Add oats, banana, and tahini, and you get a balanced smoothie that feels like a treat and will keep you satisfied.

1/2 cup frozen organic blueberries

1/4 cup rolled oats

1 cup packed baby spinach

1/2 ripe banana

1 tablespoon unsalted tahini

1/2 ripe pear, peeled, cored, and chopped (or another 1/2 banana)

1 cup unsweetened almond milk or milk of choice

Pinch of fine sea salt

TROPICAL SMOOTHIE

The flavors in this smoothie will take you away on a beach vacation right in your kitchen—plus, ginger can settle your stomach. If you're late in pregnancy, reach for this one; pineapple contains an enzyme that may help soften the cervix and has long been used as a folk remedy to encourage labor. (But don't worry, it won't induce you too early.)

1 ripe banana

1/2 cup chopped mango

1/2 cup chopped pineapple

3 tablespoons fresh orange juice

1 tablespoon hempseed hearts

1 scoop vanilla protein powder

1 teaspoon grated fresh ginger

Pinch of fine sea salt

3 ice cubes

1/2 to 1 cup unsweetened coconut milk or milk of choice

Roasted Red Pepper and Asparagus Frittata

PREP TIME: 10 MINUTES | COOK TIME: 30 MINUTES | YIELD: 4 SERVINGS

Frittatas tick all the boxes: they're simple to make, loaded with protein, flexible (they're a great way to use up stray leftover vegetables, cheese, and/or herbs), and perfect any time of day, hot or cold. Serve with a salad or potatoes for a heartier meal—or just grab a slice when you need a quick bite. Frittatas will keep covered in the fridge for up to three days. Make sure to use a skillet with an ovenproof handle.

8 large eggs

¼ cup heavy cream or canned full-fat coconut milk

2 teaspoons kosher salt, divided

Freshly ground black pepper

3 tablespoons extra-virgin olive oil

1 pound asparagus, woody ends trimmed off, thinly sliced (about 2 cups)

½ yellow onion, chopped

1 shallot, chopped

1 jarred roasted red bell pepper, patted dry and sliced (about ½ cup)

2 cups packed baby spinach

2 garlic cloves, minced

8 fresh basil leaves, thinly sliced

6 ounces soft goat cheese

1. Preheat the oven to 350°F.

2. In a large bowl, whisk together the eggs, cream, 1 teaspoon of salt, and pepper to taste.

RECIPE CONTINUES

3. In a 9-inch ovenproof skillet, warm 1 tablespoon of the oil over medium heat. Add the asparagus and sprinkle with the remaining teaspoon of salt. Cook, stirring occasionally, until tender, about 5 minutes. Transfer to a medium bowl.

4. Swirl another 1 tablespoon of oil in the skillet. Add the onion and shallot; sauté until the onion has softened, about 3 minutes. Add the roasted pepper, spinach, and garlic; cook, stirring, until the spinach has wilted and the garlic is fragrant, 1 to 2 minutes.

5. Add the asparagus back to the skillet and swirl in the last tablespoon of oil. Pour the egg mixture into the skillet; sprinkle the basil and goat cheese on top. With a spoon, lightly stir the basil and cheese into the egg mixture. Cook on the stove until the edges begin to set, about 3 minutes.

6. Transfer the skillet to the oven and cook until lightly puffed and set in the center, 12 to 15 minutes. Let the frittata cool in the pan for 5 minutes before cutting it into wedges and serving (the frittata will deflate as it cools). Alternatively, let the wedges cool completely, then wrap and refrigerate to serve later.

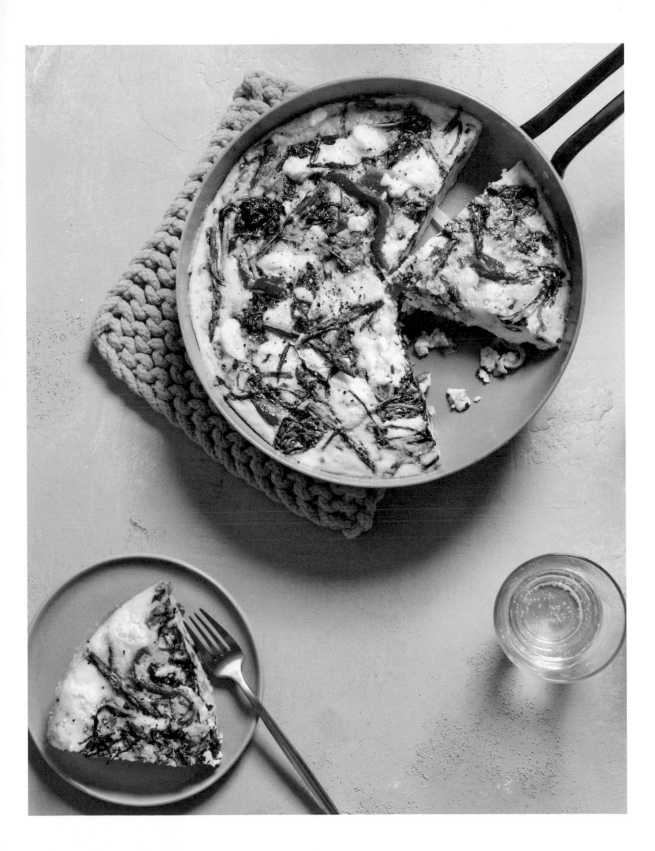

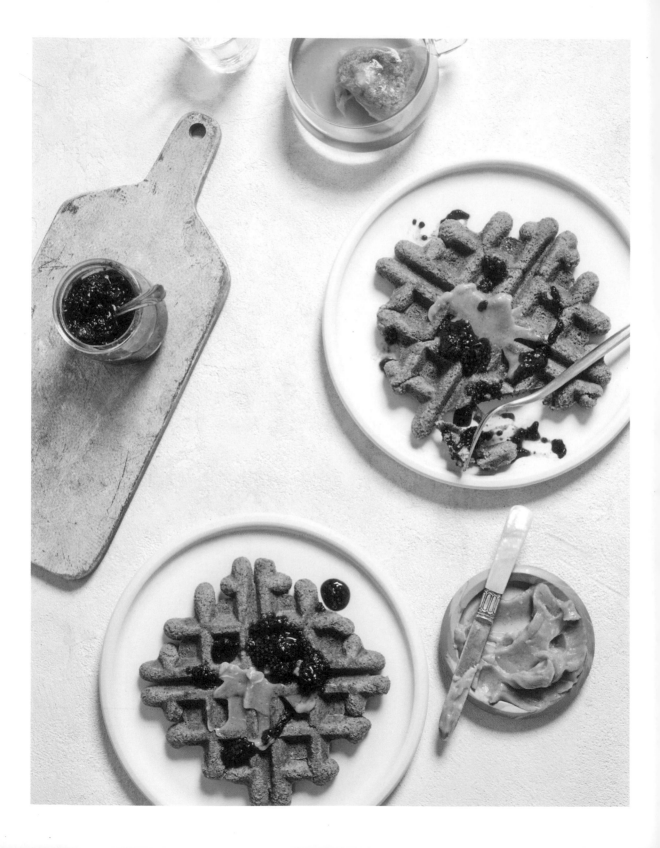

Spinach Waffles

PREP TIME: 5 MINUTES | COOK TIME: 10 TO 15 MINUTES |
YIELD: ABOUT 3 CUPS OF BATTER (ROUGHLY 6 WAFFLES DEPENDING ON
THE WAFFLE MAKER)

Who doesn't love waffles for breakfast? These are a fun and tasty way to sneak in good nutrition, with spinach, ground flaxseed, eggs, and almond flour. Make them ahead and freeze them, so all you have to do on busy mornings is pop one in the toaster oven. Kids love them too.

1 cup milk of choice

2 large eggs

½ teaspoon vanilla extract

¼ cup coconut sugar

¼ cup ghee, coconut oil, or (½ stick) unsalted butter, melted and cooled (or use a liquid fat like avocado oil or extra-virgin olive oil)

1 cup packed baby spinach

2¼ cups almond flour

¼ cup ground flaxseed

¼ teaspoon fine sea salt

½ teaspoon baking powder

½ teaspoon baking soda

Cooking spray

Cinnamon Honey Butter or Blueberry and Date Chia Jam (recipe follows)

1. Preheat the waffle iron. In a blender or food processor, combine all the ingredients except the cooking spray; blend until smooth. The batter will be thick.

2. Mist the waffle iron with cooking spray. Portion about ½ cup of batter into it and cook according to the manufacturer's instructions. Repeat with the remaining batter, misting the iron with cooking spray between batches. Serve the waffles with Cinnamon Honey Butter and Blueberry and Date Chia Jam as toppings, if desired.

RECIPE CONTINUES

at these get dark at the highest setting on my waffle iron. Lowering the heat
ngs below the highest seems to work the best for me, so you might have to
nt to find the ideal temperature.

you want to keep your waffles warm while you cook the rest, preheat the oven to
200°F. Place the cooked waffles directly on the oven rack to keep them warm and
crisp until breakfast is served.

Let any leftovers cool completely, then wrap and refrigerate or freeze. Reheat in a
toaster oven.

CINNAMON HONEY BUTTER

PREP TIME: 5 MINUTES | YIELD: ABOUT 1/4 CUP

4 tablespoons unsalted butter, at room temperature

2 tablespoons raw honey

1/2 teaspoon cinnamon

1/8 teaspoon fine sea salt

In a small bowl, combine all the ingredients and mash with a fork until
well combined. Add more cinnamon to taste. Serve right away or cover
and refrigerate to serve cold.

BLUEBERRY AND DATE CHIA JAM

PREP TIME: 2 MINUTES | COOK TIME: 10 TO 15 MINUTES | YIELD: 1 1/2 CUPS

Chia seeds are tiny powerhouses of nutrition, packed with antioxidants,
vitamins, and minerals. Plus, their unique gelling ability means you can
use them to make spreads without the piles of sugar used in traditional
jams. Chia seeds have protein and fiber, so they're great for pregnancy.
Use any in-season berries or combine the various bags of frozen ones
bumping around in your freezer. Enjoy this jam on toast, waffles,
pancakes, or oatmeal, or stir a spoonful into plain yogurt or cottage
cheese.

3 cups frozen organic blueberries

4 dried Medjool dates, pitted and finely chopped

RECIPE CONTINUES

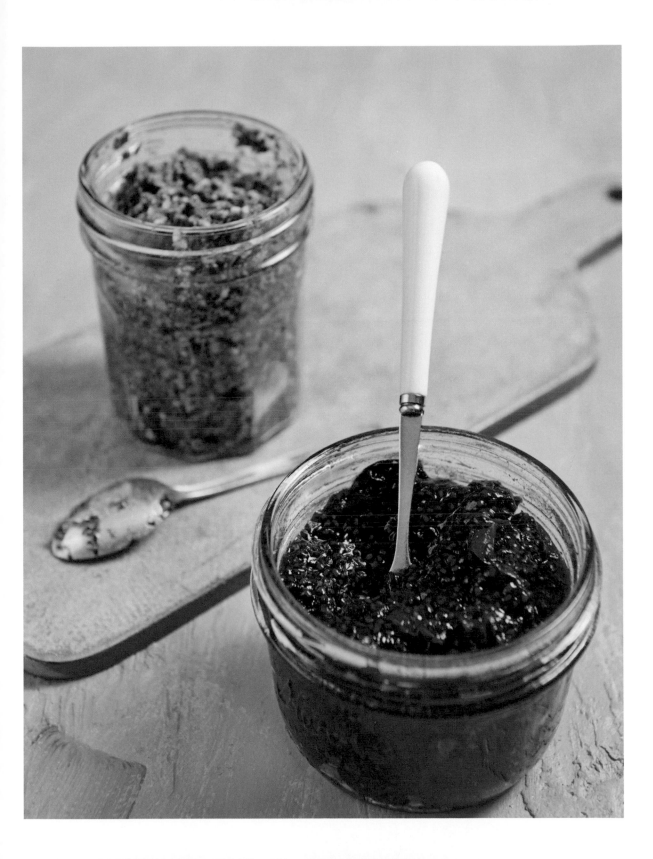

$^1/_2$ cup water

$^1/_2$ teaspoon kosher salt

Juice of $^1/_2$ medium orange (about $^1/_4$ cup)

$1^1/_2$ tablespoons fresh lemon juice

1 tablespoon maple syrup, plus more to taste

$^1/_4$ cup chia seeds

1. In a medium saucepan, combine the blueberries, dates, water, salt, both juices, and maple syrup. Place over medium heat and bring to a simmer, stirring occasionally, for about 5 minutes. Increase the heat to medium-high and lightly press the berries with the back of a spoon to help them break down.

2. Reduce the heat to medium-low and simmer, stirring occasionally, until the berries have burst and the liquid has reduced, 6 to 8 minutes.

3. Stir in the chia seeds. Cook, stirring constantly, until the chia seeds are well incorporated, about 1 minute. Remove the pan from the heat; let cool for 5 minutes. Stir in up to an additional tablespoon of maple syrup to taste. Let cool completely, stirring occasionally.

4. Transfer the jam to a clean bowl or jar, cover, and refrigerate. It will keep for up to 2 weeks or may be frozen for up to 2 months.

NOTES

Feel free to swap in another berry, or use a combination.

Use honey in place of maple syrup, if you prefer.

Try adding other flavors to your jam. Stir in ground cinnamon or ginger during the cooking time, or add a little vanilla extract after taking the jam off the heat.

Quinoa and Veggie Breakfast Bowl

PREP TIME: 15 MINUTES | COOK TIME: 20 MINUTES | YIELD: 4 SERVINGS

Sometimes you need something super hearty and filling to start your day. Feel free to omit the bacon and eggs or scramble a couple of eggs with the quinoa when you reheat. These bowls are full of savory, healthy fats and bright, citrusy arugula to keep them from feeling heavy. I love the combination of zucchini and mushrooms, but feel free to clean your fridge out and sneak in any veggies you find.

4 slices thick-cut bacon or 4 break-fast sausages

4 eggs

2 tablespoons (¼ stick) unsalted butter or high-heat oil of choice

½ medium red onion, finely diced (about 1 cup)

1 clove garlic, grated or minced

1 teaspoon kosher salt, plus more to taste

Freshly ground black pepper

1 medium zucchini, finely diced

12 small to medium cremini mushrooms

2 cups cooked quinoa or grain of choice

3 cups packed arugula

¼ to ⅓ cup fresh, thinly sliced basil

2 teaspoons fresh lemon juice

1 avocado, flesh scooped and sliced

Crumbled feta

1. Prepare your bacon and eggs (this can be done ahead of time): Cook the bacon (or sausage) according to the package directions. While the bacon is cooking, bring a large pot of water to a boil. Using a slotted spoon, carefully lower the eggs into the boiling water, and reduce the heat slightly. Boil for 7 minutes, then immediately transfer to an ice bath to stop the cooking. Let the eggs cool, then peel. Set aside the bacon and eggs while you prepare the rest of the ingredients.

RECIPE CONTINUES

2. In a large skillet, melt the butter over medium heat. Add the red onion, garlic, $\frac{1}{2}$ teaspoon of the salt, and pepper to taste. Sauté for 3 minutes.

3. Add the zucchini and mushrooms and another $\frac{1}{2}$ teaspoon of salt. Sauté for 6 to 7 minutes until the zucchini is tender and the mushrooms are wilted and soft.

4. To the same pan, dump in the quinoa and stir, letting the quinoa warm. Transfer everything in the pan to a large bowl. Add the arugula and basil and toss to combine, letting the arugula slightly wilt from the residual heat. Pour in the lemon juice and add salt and pepper to taste.

5. To serve: Add a quarter of the quinoa mixture to a bowl and top with a quarter of the avocado slices, crumbled feta, and bacon and one jammy egg. Portion the rest into glass containers, stored in the fridge, to enjoy the rest of the week.

BAKED GOODS

Homemade Granola Bars

PREP TIME: 15 MINUTES | COOK TIME: 25 TO 30 MINUTES | YIELD: 16 BARS

Granola bars can be super healthy or junky sugar bombs. Rather than rolling the dice with a packaged brand, whip up your own. It's as easy as tossing together a few pantry items and baking, and you can change up the ingredients to suit your tastes. Swap in different nuts and seeds, use whatever nut butter you have on hand, mix up the spices—make them your own. You'll be happy to have a snack that you can easily munch on with one hand while you're holding the baby with the other.

Cooking spray (preferably olive or avocado oil)

¾ cup finely chopped pecans

½ cup raw pumpkin seeds

¼ cup hempseed hearts

¼ cup roasted, lightly salted sunflower seeds

¾ cup unsweetened shredded coconut

⅓ cup smooth, runny nut or seed butter (such as almond butter, tahini, or mixed-nut butter)

⅓ cup raw honey

1 teaspoon vanilla extract

½ teaspoon cinnamon

¼ teaspoon fine sea salt (optional)

1. Preheat the oven to 325°F. Line an 8 × 8-inch baking dish with parchment paper, allowing it to overlap the edges of the baking dish on two sides; lightly mist the parchment with cooking spray.

RECIPE CONTINUES

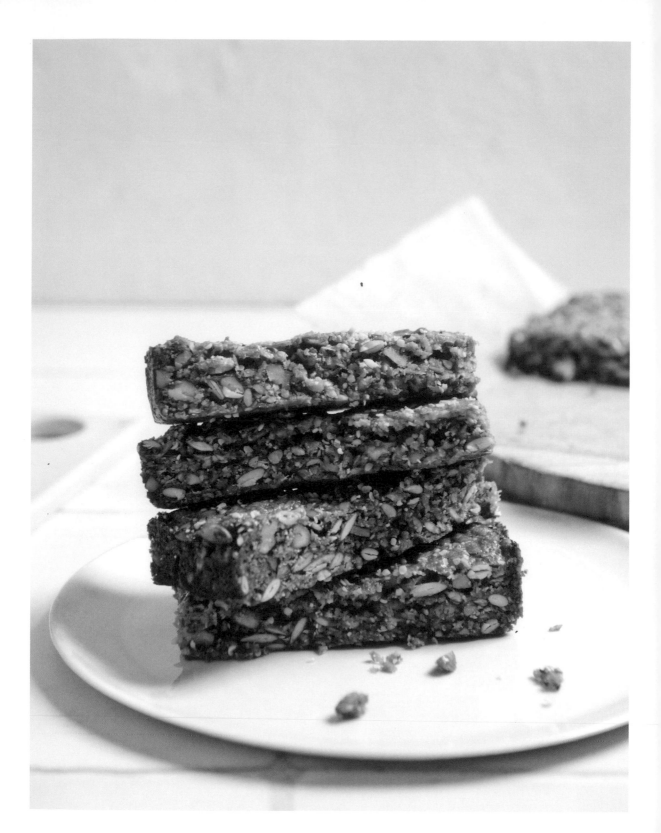

2. In a large bowl, combine the pecans, pumpkin seeds, hempseed hearts, sunflower seeds, and coconut, tossing to mix well. In a small saucepan, combine the nut butter and honey. Place over low heat and cook, stirring, until the mixture is just warmed through and well mixed, 1 to 2 minutes. Remove from the heat and stir in the vanilla, cinnamon, and salt, if using. Stir the nut butter mixture into the nut and seed mixture until all the ingredients are well combined (the mixture will be very thick and sticky).

3. Spread the mixture into the baking dish, pressing it into an even layer. Bake until golden, 25 to 30 minutes. Transfer the pan to a wire rack to cool completely.

4. Remove the baked granola from the pan using the parchment paper as a handle. Peel off the parchment paper. Using a sharp knife, cut into 16 pieces. Keep leftovers covered in the refrigerator for up to 1 week.

NOTE

Check the label of your nut butter to see if it's salted; if so, you can omit the optional salt.

rrot Cake Muffins

Dessert for breakfast? Why not, when it's a grain- and refined sugar–free carrot cake muffin. These are loaded with warming spices, yummy but not too sweet, and easy to grab on busy mornings. Top one with a little cream cheese mixed with a dab of honey if you like your carrot cake with "frosting."

1¾ cups blanched almond flour

¼ cup arrowroot flour

1½ teaspoons cinnamon

1 teaspoon ground ginger

½ teaspoon nutmeg

½ teaspoon baking soda

¼ teaspoon fine sea salt

3 large eggs

⅓ cup maple syrup

¼ cup extra-virgin olive oil

1 teaspoon vanilla extract

1 cup shredded carrots

⅓ cup finely chopped walnuts

¼ cup raisins (optional)

1. Preheat the oven to 350°F. Line a 12-cup muffin tin with paper liners.

2. In a large bowl, combine the almond flour, arrowroot, cinnamon, ginger, nutmeg, baking soda, and salt; whisk to mix well. In a medium bowl, whisk together the eggs, maple syrup, oil, and vanilla. Pour the

RECIPE CONTINUES

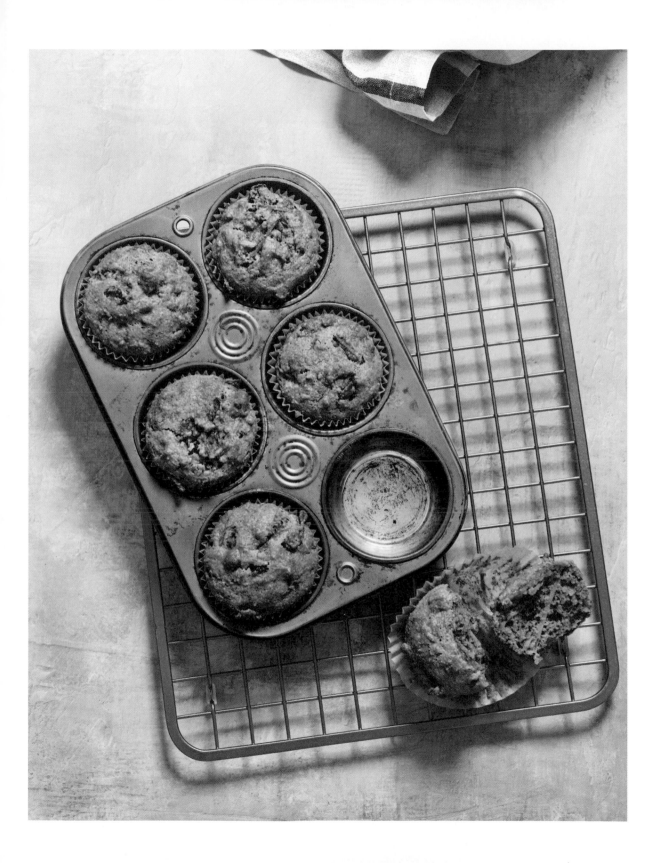

egg mixture into the flour mixture and stir until nearly combined. Fold in the carrot, walnuts, and raisins, if using.

3. Divide the batter among the muffin cups. Bake until the muffins are golden and a toothpick inserted into one comes out clean, 20 to 25 minutes. Let the muffins cool in the pan on a wire rack for 5 minutes, then transfer them to the rack to cool completely. Keep leftovers covered and refrigerated for up to 4 days.

NOTES

If you want sweeter muffins, add another tablespoon of maple syrup to the batter. Alternatively, mix 1 teaspoon of cinnamon with 1 tablespoon of coconut sugar. Brush the tops of the baked muffins with a little melted butter and sprinkle with the cinnamon-sugar mixture.

You can use 1 tablespoon of pre-made pumpkin pie or apple pie spice in place of the cinnamon, ginger, and nutmeg in the batter, if you like.

Feel free to swap chopped pecans, almonds, or pistachios for the walnuts. Unsweetened coconut flakes are also a good option.

Tahini Banana Bread

PREP TIME: 15 MINUTES | COOK TIME: 45 TO 50 MINUTES | YIELD: 1 (9-INCH) LOAF (ABOUT 8 SLICES)

A slice of homemade banana bread is so comforting, and when made strategically, it also can be a nutrient-packed snack. Tahini gives this version a rich, ever-so-slightly savory edge, and it's a good source of calcium, super important for pregnancy. This bread is also grain- and gluten-free and has no refined sugar. Enjoy a slice warm from the oven or cold from the fridge, plain or with a slather of cream cheese. Freeze a few slices for after the baby comes.

1½ cups almond flour

¼ cup arrowroot flour

¼ cup collagen peptides (or replace with almond flour)

1 teaspoon baking soda

1½ teaspoons cinnamon

¼ teaspoon fine sea salt

3 medium ripe bananas

⅓ cup tahini

¼ cup maple syrup

2 large eggs

1 teaspoon vanilla extract

OPTIONAL TOPPING

1 tablespoon coconut sugar

½ teaspoon cinnamon

1. Preheat the oven to 350°F. Line a 9 × 5-inch loaf pan with parchment paper.

2. In a large bowl, whisk together the almond flour, arrowroot, collagen, baking soda, cinnamon, and salt. In a separate, medium bowl, mash the bananas. Add the tahini, maple syrup, eggs, and vanilla; whisk until well combined. Add the tahini mixture to the almond flour mixture and stir until well combined. Transfer the batter to the loaf pan, spreading it evenly.

RECIPE CONTINUES

3. Make the topping, if using: In a cup, mix the coconut sugar and cinnamon. Sprinkle over the batter. Use a butter knife or chopstick to swirl it into a marble pattern.

4. Bake the bread until a toothpick inserted in the center comes out clean, 45 to 50 minutes (cover it with foil after 35 to 40 minutes if it starts to brown too much).

5. Let the bread cool in the pan on a wire rack for 10 minutes, then turn the bread out and let it cool completely on the rack. Keep leftovers wrapped in the fridge for up to 5 days, or slice, wrap the slices individually, and freeze for up to 3 months.

NOTES

If you have a bunch of bananas turning brown, freeze them for smoothies and future banana bread. Peel each banana and wrap it individually (I like to break it into pieces first) so you can use them easily in recipes. For baking, defrost overnight in the fridge or on the counter for 30 to 60 minutes. They'll be mushy and brown; that's okay.

You can fold in some mini chocolate chips or a finely chopped dark chocolate bar before baking.

COMFORT FOODS

Ginger Veggie Fried Rice

PREP TIME: 20 MINUTES | COOK TIME: 15 MINUTES | YIELD: 4 SERVINGS

No wonder rice is a staple in so many cuisines. It's simple and starchy, it's delicious as a main dish or side, it can take on bold flavors, or you can enjoy it with a little melted butter and salt.

For this dish, I start with cooked rice, and it's best if the rice has had time to rest in the fridge overnight as it will hold its shape better. It's also a fantastic way to use up extra rice from takeout. Follow the recipe as is, or toss in any stray vegetables you have on hand, cooked or uncooked. Feel free to add any cooked protein you like—shrimp, chicken, tofu, etc.

SAUCE

2 teaspoons toasted sesame oil

2 tablespoons unseasoned rice vinegar

3 tablespoons coconut aminos

4 garlic cloves, grated

2 teaspoons grated fresh ginger

Kosher salt and freshly ground black pepper

FRIED RICE

2½ tablespoons avocado oil

½ medium white onion, thinly sliced

RECIPE CONTINUES

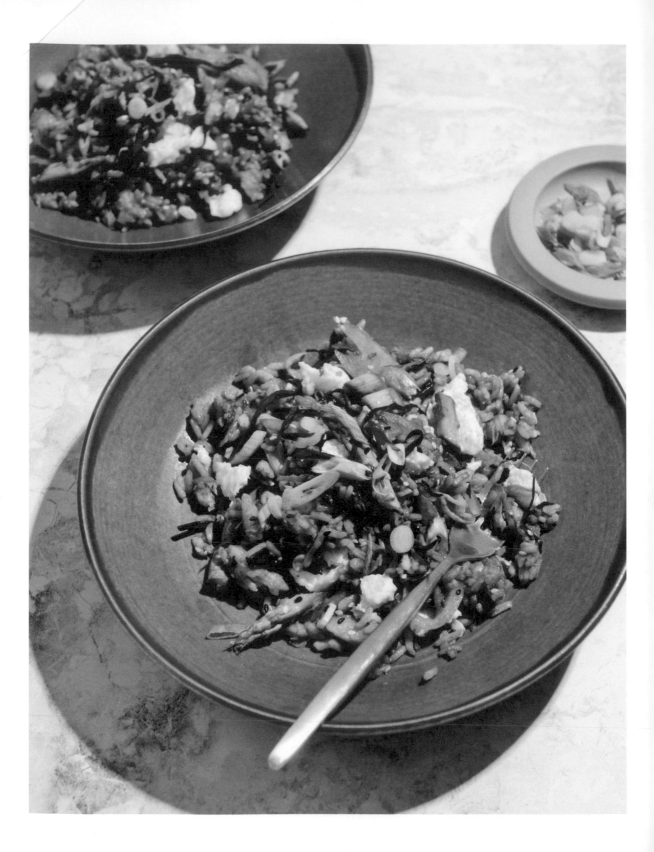

2 celery stalks, trimmed, thinly sliced on a diagonal (optional)

1 cup snap or snow peas, thinly sliced

1 teaspoon kosher salt, plus more to taste

1 bunch asparagus, woody ends trimmed, sliced ½ inch thick on a diagonal

1 cup shredded purple cabbage

3 large eggs, beaten

2 cups chilled cooked rice, preferably a day old

4 scallions (white and light green parts only), thinly sliced

2 tablespoons toasted sesame seeds

1. Make the sauce: In a small bowl, whisk together the sesame oil, vinegar, coconut aminos, garlic, and ginger. Season with salt and pepper to taste.

2. In a large skillet or wok, heat 1 tablespoon of the avocado oil over medium heat. Add the onion, optional celery, snap peas, and ½ teaspoon of the salt. Cook, stirring constantly, until the vegetables are tender but still crunchy, 3 to 5 minutes. Transfer to a large bowl.

3. In the same skillet, warm another 1 tablespoon of avocado oil. Add the asparagus and cabbage; season with the remaining ½ teaspoon of salt. Stir-fry until the vegetables are tender but not mushy, 3 to 5 minutes. Transfer to the bowl with the onion mixture.

4. In the same skillet, warm the remaining ½ tablespoon of avocado oil. Add the eggs and cook, stirring, until just beginning to set, about 1 minute.

5. Return the vegetables to the skillet with the eggs and add the rice. Pour in the sauce and add the scallions. Cook, stirring constantly, until everything is mixed well and coated with sauce, and the rice is warmed through, 2 to 3 minutes. Season with more salt to taste. Sprinkle with the sesame seeds and serve.

RECIPE CONTINUES

NOTES

If you have leftover fried rice, allow it to cool, then cover and refrigerate it for up to 3 days. For a fun way to enjoy it, reheat it in your waffle iron.

One of my favorite shortcuts is frozen grated ginger. You'll find it in many supermarkets in the freezer section, portioned into 1-teaspoon cubes. You don't even have to defrost it; just toss it into whatever you're cooking.

Breaded Chicken Cutlets with Pickle-y Slaw

PREP TIME: 15 MINUTES | MARINATE TIME: OVERNIGHT |
COOK TIME: 25 MINUTES | YIELD: 6 SERVINGS (1 CUTLET EACH)

If ever there was a pregnancy comfort food recipe, this is it! Breaded chicken with pickled slaw, c'mon! Use these cutlets in sandwiches, slice and toss them on a salad, drizzle them with a sauce of your choosing, or enjoy them on their own whenever you've got a craving for a crunchy, high-protein bite. They will keep covered in the fridge for up to three days, or wrap well and freeze for up to six months. They pair delectably with the slaw for a mouthwatering way to satisfy those cravings.

CHICKEN

2 tablespoons extra-virgin olive oil

1 teaspoon grated lemon zest

1 teaspoon fresh lemon juice

2 teaspoons salt

2 tablespoons plus 1 teaspoon dried thyme

1 tablespoon plus 1 teaspoon Dijon mustard

2 pounds boneless, skinless chicken breast, cut into 6 pieces and pounded to ¼-inch thickness (see notes)

3 large eggs, beaten

1 teaspoon garlic powder

1½ cups panko bread crumbs (or gluten-free panko)

¼ cup freshly grated Parmesan

Cooking spray (preferably olive or avocado oil)

RECIPE CONTINUES

SLAW

4 cups shredded green or purple cabbage

½ red onion, thinly sliced

1 (24-ounce) jar sweet bread-and-butter pickles, roughly chopped or sliced, juice reserved

1 tablespoon apple cider vinegar

Kosher salt and freshly ground black pepper, to taste

1. In a small bowl, whisk together the oil, lemon zest, lemon juice, 1 teaspoon of salt, 2 tablespoons of thyme, and 1 tablespoon of mustard.

2. Rub the mixture over the chicken breasts. Place the chicken in a zipper bag and refrigerate overnight.

3. Preheat the oven to 400°F. Line a rimmed baking sheet with parchment paper.

4. Make the slaw: In a large bowl, place the cabbage and onions. Add the pickles and their juice, vinegar, and salt and pepper to taste; toss to combine. Let sit at room temperature for at least 30 minutes. The slaw will be ready after 30 minutes but will continue to develop flavor as it sits.

5. Make the chicken: In a medium bowl, whisk together the eggs, 1 teaspoon of mustard, 1 teaspoon of salt, and the garlic powder.

6. On a plate or in a shallow pan, whisk together the bread crumbs and the Parmesan.

7. Wipe any excess marinade from the cutlets with a paper towel.

8. Dip each cutlet first in the egg mixture and then in the bread crumb mixture to coat. Set on the prepared baking sheet.

9. Spray the cutlets with the cooking spray.

10. Bake until the chicken is browned, 15 minutes. Flip the cutlets. Continue to cook until the second sides are browned, 8 to 10 minutes more.

11. The slaw can be placed on the chicken or used as a side dish.

AIR FRYER INSTRUCTIONS

1. Follow instructions 1 through 8 above, preheating your air fryer instead of your oven.
2. Spritz the inside of the air fryer with the cooking spray.
3. Place the chicken into the air fryer in a single layer. Cook for 15 minutes, flipping after 7½ minutes.

NOTES

To save time, you can omit the first step and not marinate the chicken.

To pound out the cutlets, place them between two pieces of parchment paper or plastic wrap. Use a kitchen mallet (or even the side of a can of food) to evenly pound them to the desired thickness. If you have a favorite local butcher, you can ask them to slice your chicken breast thinly to be used for this recipe.

If acid reflux is an issue, you may want to omit the raw onions from the slaw.

Beef and Broccoli

PREP TIME: 15 MINUTES | MARINATE TIME: 15 MINUTES |
COOK TIME: 15 MINUTES | YIELD: 4 SERVINGS

Tender and thinly sliced marinated beef pairs with crunchy broccoli in this flavorful recipe. You can throw it together in the time it takes to order takeout and get it delivered, and this version is lighter and healthier. Serve it with Super-Simple Ginger Slaw (page 227) for a vegetable-packed meal or on top of rice or noodles to soak up all the tasty sauce.

1¼ pounds sirloin steak

¾ cup coconut aminos

3 tablespoons unseasoned rice vinegar

1½ teaspoons toasted sesame oil

1 teaspoon grated fresh ginger

3 garlic cloves, grated

1 teaspoon raw honey

2 teaspoons kosher salt

¼ teaspoon freshly ground black pepper

2 teaspoons tapioca starch or arrowroot flour

3 tablespoons avocado oil

1 pound broccoli florets, cut into bite-sized pieces

1 small white onion, thinly sliced

½ cup fresh basil leaves

4 scallions (white and light green parts only), thinly sliced

1½ tablespoons toasted sesame seeds

1. Place the steak in the freezer while you prepare the ingredients for the marinade (this will make the beef easier to slice).

2. In a large bowl, whisk together the coconut aminos, vinegar, sesame oil, ginger, garlic, honey, salt, and pepper. In a separate small bowl, mix the tapioca starch with 2 teaspoons of water, stirring until dissolved.

3. Remove the steak from the freezer; place it on a cutting board. Using a sharp chef's knife, thinly slice it against the grain. Add to the bowl with the marinade and toss to combine. Let it stand for at least 15 minutes or up to 1 hour.

4. In a large skillet or wok, warm 2 tablespoons of the avocado oil over high heat. Add the broccoli and sauté until tender but still crunchy and caramelized in spots, 6 to 7 minutes. Transfer the broccoli to a large bowl.

5. Reduce the heat to medium. In the same skillet, warm the remaining 1 tablespoon of avocado oil. Add the onions; sauté until softened, 2 minutes. Using tongs, remove the steak from the marinade and add it to the skillet, reserving the marinade. Sauté the steak and onions until almost cooked through, about 2 minutes. Pour the marinade into the skillet. Stir the tapioca starch mixture, then add it to the skillet. Reduce the heat and simmer, stirring occasionally, until the sauce thickens, about 1 minute.

6. Once the sauce has thickened, add the broccoli and basil leaves to the skillet and toss to combine. Divide among four plates or shallow bowls, top with the scallions and sesame seeds, and serve.

NOTE

You can swap in another protein here. Try thinly sliced boneless pork chops or chicken breasts, or medium shrimp.

Everything Bagel Popcorn

PREP TIME: 1 MINUTE | COOK TIME: 15 MINUTES | YIELD: ABOUT 13 CUPS, POPPED

We're so used to microwave popcorn, the idea of making it fresh on the stove seems complicated. But it's actually really simple, and healthier than most microwave varieties, which are often made with additives and lower-quality kernels. Shake up the classic salt and butter combo with everything bagel seasoning blend. Nutritional yeast or grated Parmesan also works well.

3 tablespoons avocado or coconut oil

½ cup popcorn kernels

4 tablespoons unsalted butter

2 tablespoons everything bagel seasoning

Kosher salt

1. In a large heavy-bottomed pot, warm the oil over medium-high heat for about 30 seconds. Add the kernels, cover the pot, and cook, gently shaking the pot. You'll hear the kernels popping; keep shaking occasionally. Once the popping slows (1 to 2 seconds between pops), uncover and transfer the popcorn to two large bowls.

2. Let the pot cool slightly, and carefully wipe out the remnants with a paper towel. Return the pot to the stove over low heat and add the butter. Once the butter has melted, add the everything bagel seasoning.

3. Divide the butter mixture between the two bowls of popcorn and toss with utensils to combine. Season with additional salt to taste. Serve right away. Store leftovers in an airtight container at room temperature for up to 4 days.

NOTE

Everything bagel seasoning varies among brands, and some are saltier than others. Taste your popcorn before adding more salt.

VEGGIES

Marinated Cucumber Two Ways

PREP TIME: 10 MINUTES | YIELD: 4 TO 6 SERVINGS

Crunchy and cold, refreshing and hydrating, marinated cucumbers are a delicious and easy way to get in your nutrition, even when plain vegetables don't feel appealing. Enjoy them as a side dish, toss them into a salad, or pat them dry and use as a topping for your favorite sandwich. English cucumbers are the simplest, with their thin skin, but if they aren't available, use regular cucumbers (just peel them). Persian cucumbers are also a good option; they're thin-skinned like English, but smaller, so you can eat a whole one in one go—I lived on them during both of my pregnancies.

JAPANESE-INSPIRED VERSION

2 English cucumbers, ends trimmed, thinly sliced

1 tablespoon coconut aminos

¾ cup unseasoned rice vinegar

2 tablespoons water

2 tablespoons olive or avocado oil

¼ teaspoon toasted sesame oil

2 teaspoons toasted sesame seeds

SIMPLE MARINATED CUCUMBERS

2 English cucumbers, ends trimmed, thinly sliced

¼ cup apple cider vinegar

RECIPE CONTINUES

¼ cup unseasoned rice vinegar

¼ cup extra-virgin olive oil

½ teaspoon kosher salt

Freshly ground black pepper

For both options: In a large bowl, combine all the ingredients. Cover and refrigerate for at least 1 hour, stirring occasionally. Keep covered and refrigerated for up to 3 days.

Butternut Squash and Apple Soup

PREP TIME: 30 MINUTES | COOK TIME: 45 TO 55 MINUTES | YIELD: ABOUT 11 CUPS

Soup is the ultimate comfort food, warming, soothing, and easy on the belly. This one is jam-packed with optimal nutrition, thanks to the apples, vegetables, garlic, and spices, all of which really bring the flavor. Sip it on its own, have a cup with a sandwich for lunch, or stir in some cooked grains to add bulk. This recipe yields a lot; freeze a few portions in single-serve containers for up to three months (be sure to leave some space at the top, as liquid expands when it freezes).

¼ cup oil (extra-virgin olive, avocado, or coconut)

1 medium yellow onion, chopped (about 1½ cups)

3 celery stalks, trimmed and sliced ¼ inch thick (about 1 cup)

2 large carrots, chopped

5 teaspoons kosher salt

½ teaspoon freshly ground black pepper, plus more to taste

6 garlic cloves, minced (about 2 tablespoons)

1 tablespoon ground coriander

1 teaspoon smoked paprika

2 small or 1 large butternut squash, trimmed, peeled, seeded, and cut into 1½-inch chunks

2 sweet apples, such as Fuji or Gala, peeled, cored, and chopped

4 cups low-sodium chicken bone broth, mixed with 2 cups water

3 fresh thyme sprigs

1 (13.5-ounce) can full-fat coconut milk

1 tablespoon apple cider vinegar

RECIPE CONTINUES

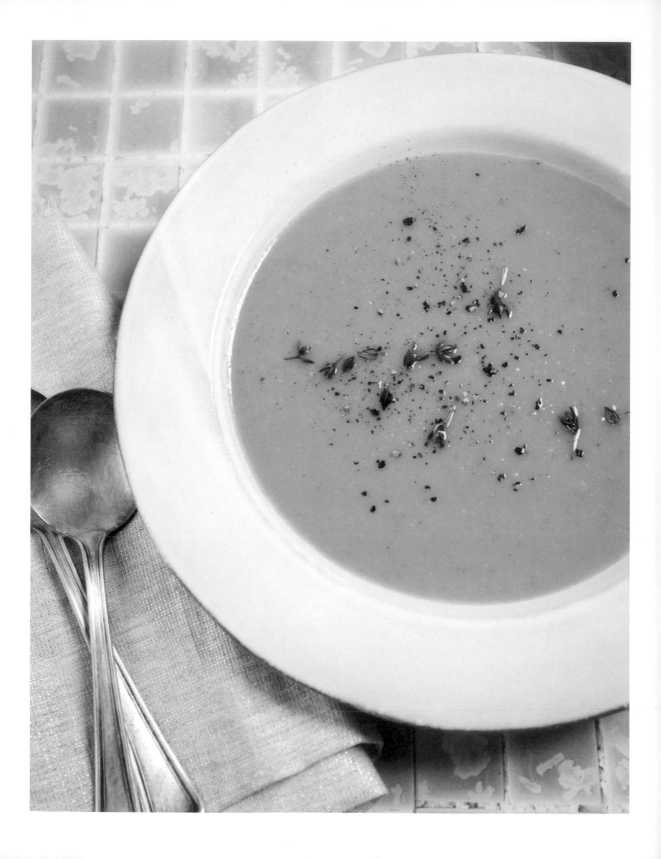

1. In a large heavy-bottomed pot, warm the oil over medium heat. Add the onions, celery, and carrots, season with 1 teaspoon of the salt and the pepper and cook, stirring occasionally, until the vegetables are tender and the onions begin to become translucent, 5 to 6 minutes. Add the garlic, coriander, and smoked paprika; cook, stirring, until fragrant, 30 seconds to 1 minute.

2. Add the squash, apples, broth, and thyme; stir in 3 teaspoons of the salt. If the vegetables aren't covered, add water half a cup at a time (up to 2 cups) until they are, raise the heat to high, bring the soup to a boil, then reduce the heat to medium.

3. Simmer the mixture until the squash is very tender, 40 to 50 minutes. Turn off the heat. Using tongs, remove and discard the thyme sprigs. Stir in the coconut milk and vinegar.

4. Using an immersion blender, blend the soup until silky and creamy and no lumps remain. (Alternatively, transfer to a high-speed blender to blend.) Season with the remaining 1 teaspoon of salt and additional pepper to taste. Serve right away or let cool completely, cover, and refrigerate for up to 5 days.

NOTE

This soup will taste even better after sitting around for a while. If you have the time, make it a day ahead, let it cool completely, then cover and refrigerate. Rewarm it gently over medium-low heat the next day.

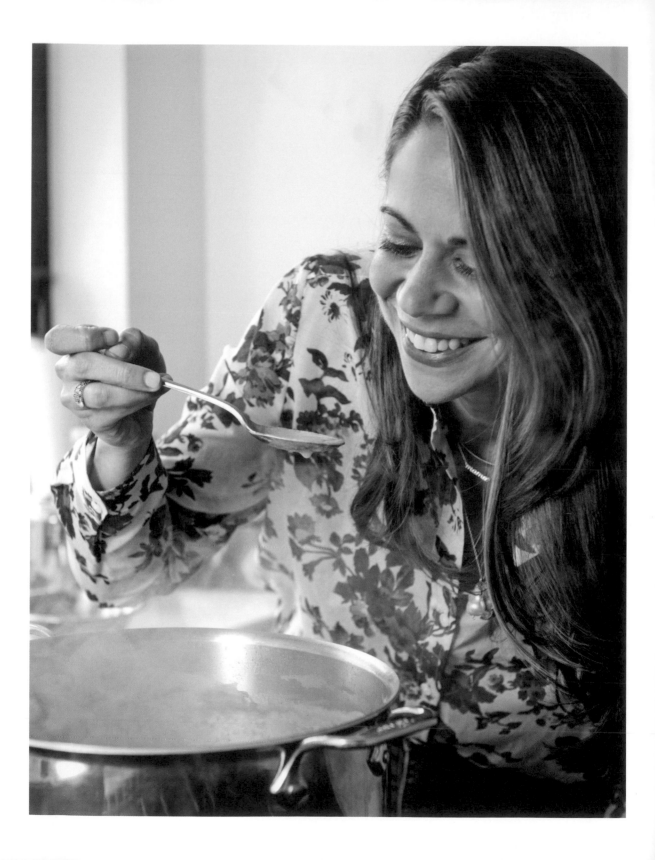

Super-Simple Ginger Slaw

A good slaw is a gift: it's a refreshing and flavorful way to get loads of vegetables in, the zingy vinegar base satisfies those pickle cravings, and it holds up well for a few days in the fridge. This one also includes fresh ginger, which can be soothing to the stomach. Enjoy it as a side dish or make it the main event by topping it with a cooked protein, like chicken or shrimp and/or a scattering of chopped toasted nuts.

DRESSING

2 tablespoons extra-virgin olive oil

1 teaspoon toasted sesame oil

¼ cup unseasoned rice vinegar

2 tablespoons coconut aminos or tamari

1½ teaspoons raw honey

1 clove garlic, grated

1 teaspoon grated fresh ginger

Kosher salt and freshly ground black pepper

SLAW

1 red bell pepper, seeded and thinly sliced (about 2 cups)

2 cups shredded green cabbage

2 cups shredded red cabbage

1 cup shredded carrots (about 2 to 3 medium carrots)

4 scallions (white and light green parts only), thinly sliced on a diagonal

Kosher salt and freshly ground black pepper

1½ tablespoons toasted sesame seeds

RECIPE CONTINUES

1. Make the dressing: In a jar with a tight-fitting lid, combine all the ingredients except the salt and pepper. Cover tightly and shake until well combined and emulsified. Season with salt and pepper to taste.

2. Make the slaw: In a large bowl, combine all the ingredients except the sesame seeds; toss to mix. Add the dressing and toss to combine. Season with additional salt and pepper to taste. Sprinkle with sesame seeds and serve.

NOTE

Make this easy dish even easier by using a couple of bags of premade coleslaw mix instead of shredding the cabbage and carrots.

Spinach and Pistachio Pesto

PREP TIME: 10 MINUTES | YIELD: 1 CUP

Basil and pine nut pesto is a classic combo for a reason—and this version, which brings together pistachios and spinach, hits those same notes with a fresh, elegant twist. Bonus: spinach is an excellent source of folate, an important nutrient for a healthy pregnancy. The addition of the ice cube is a trick to keep the pesto bright and green. Toss this with any pasta or grain, use it to top protein or veggies, or spoon it over a pizza.

2 cups packed baby spinach

1 cup packed whole fresh basil leaves

¾ cup roasted shelled pistachios

2 tablespoons fresh lemon juice

½ cup freshly grated Parmesan

1 clove garlic, smashed

½ cup extra-virgin olive oil, plus more to cover

1 ice cube

Kosher salt

In a high-powered blender or food processor, combine the spinach, basil, pistachios, lemon juice, Parmesan, and garlic; pulse to mix and roughly chop. With the machine running, slowly drizzle in the oil until the mixture is very finely chopped and well combined. Add the ice cube and process until completely mixed in, scraping down the sides of the blender as needed. Season with salt to taste. Transfer to an airtight container, top with just enough oil to cover the surface, cover, and refrigerate for up to 5 days.

NOTE

You can save this pesto, and you will be glad you did. Add portions to an ice cube tray and freeze, then transfer the cubes to a silicone bag to keep for up to 6 months in the freezer.

Winter Squash Salad

PREP TIME: 15 MINUTES | COOK TIME: 25 TO 30 MINUTES | YIELD: 4 TO 6 SERVINGS

When I was pregnant with my second baby, I craved this one kale salad from a café near my apartment so often, I had to create my own. With most salads, you have to eat them right after tossing with the dressing, or they get soggy. But this one lasts for a few days covered in the fridge, so you can have it as a quick meal on a busy day or just to nosh when you want immediate satisfaction. It's delectable on its own, or you can add additional protein like hard-cooked eggs or leftover chicken. I use delicata squash because you don't have to peel it, but you can swap in butternut, acorn, or another variety.

VINAIGRETTE

1½ teaspoons Dijon mustard

¼ cup plus 2 tablespoons red wine vinegar

¾ cup extra-virgin olive oil

Kosher salt and freshly ground black pepper

SALAD

2 medium to large delicata squash, trimmed, halved lengthwise, seeds removed, sliced ½ inch thick

2 tablespoons avocado oil

½ teaspoon garlic powder

½ teaspoon onion powder

2 teaspoons kosher salt

¼ teaspoon freshly ground black pepper

1 bunch dinosaur kale, ribs removed, leaves sliced into thin ribbons

1 teaspoon extra-virgin olive oil

1 (14-ounce) can white beans (cannellini or great northern), drained and rinsed

RECIPE CONTINUES

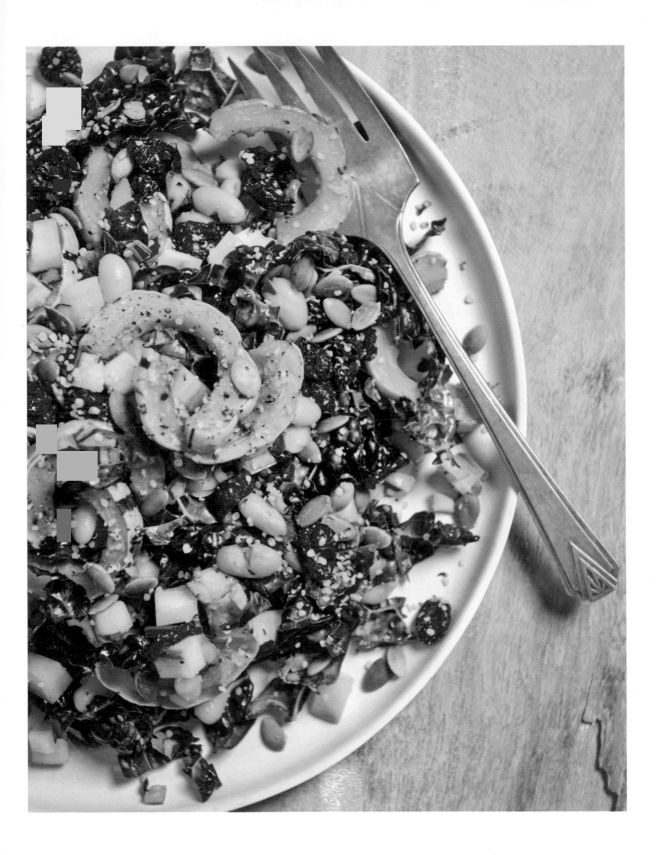

1 English cucumber, diced

1 small red onion, finely diced

⅓ cup dried cranberries

⅓ cup toasted pumpkin seeds

Kosher salt and freshly ground black pepper

1. Preheat the oven to 425°F. Line a large baking sheet with parchment paper.

2. Make the vinaigrette: In a small jar, combine the mustard, vinegar, and oil. Cover and shake vigorously until well mixed and emulsified. Season with salt and pepper to taste.

3. Place the squash in a large bowl. Add the avocado oil, garlic powder, onion powder, 1½ teaspoons of the salt, and the pepper; toss to combine. Spread the squash into a single layer on the prepared baking sheet. Roast until the squash is tender and caramelized in spots, 25 to 30 minutes, turning over halfway through. Transfer the baking sheet to a wire rack and let the squash cool.

4. Place the kale in the same large bowl. Drizzle with the olive oil and sprinkle with the remaining ½ teaspoon of salt. Using your hands, scrunch and massage the kale until it softens and relaxes, 30 seconds to 1 minute. Add the beans, cucumber, red onions, cranberries, pumpkin seeds, and cooled squash to the bowl. Add 3 tablespoons of the dressing; toss to coat (add in more of the dressing, if desired). Season the salad with additional salt and pepper to taste.

NOTES

Don't discard those kale stems. Slice and add them to a stir-fry or soup, or chop and freeze them to add to smoothies.

If you find raw onion hard to digest, halve and thinly slice the onion and roast it along with the squash, then toss it into the salad with the other add-ins. Or just leave it out.

Swap chickpeas for white beans, if you prefer.

Crispy Baked Sweet Potato Fries

PREP TIME: 20 MINUTES | SOAK TIME: 30 MINUTES |
COOK TIME: 20 MINUTES | YIELD: 4 SERVINGS

When you're craving fries, nothing else will hit the spot. With this recipe, you can scratch that itch with nourishment and no mess. The starch helps the fries crisp without having to use a ton of oil. Enjoy them as a side dish or share them at snack time. In the unlikely event that you have leftovers, reheat them in a 350°F oven or for a few minutes in the air fryer.

4 small sweet potatoes, scrubbed and dried

4 tablespoons avocado oil

2 tablespoons cornstarch

2 teaspoons garlic powder

1 teaspoon onion powder

1 teaspoon kosher salt

Freshly ground black pepper

1. Trim off the ends of the sweet potatoes, then halve them lengthwise. Slightly angle the knife and cut each half into wedges (you should get 4 to 6 out of each half, or 8 to 12 per potato). Place the wedges in a large bowl of cold water and allow them to soak for 30 minutes to 1 hour to remove the starch. Preheat the oven to 450°F.

2. Drain the potatoes, pat them dry thoroughly, and transfer them to a large bowl. Line two baking sheets with parchment paper. Brush 2 tablespoons of oil over each baking sheet.

3. Sprinkle the sweet potatoes with the cornstarch, garlic powder, onion powder, and salt; season with pepper. Toss to combine. Shake off any excess cornstarch mixture and divide the wedges between the prepared

RECIPE CONTINUES

baking sheets, spreading them into a single layer and making sure they don't touch.

4. Bake until the fries are golden and crisp, about 20 minutes, flipping halfway through. Serve hot.

SHEET PANS AND BOWLS

Sheet Pan Miso Salmon and Bok Choy

PREP TIME: 15 MINUTES | COOK TIME: 15 MINUTES | YIELD: 4 SERVINGS

Low in mercury and high in healthy omega-3 fats, salmon is a prime fish option for pregnancy, and a one-sheet-pan meal means hassle-free cleanup. Wild-caught salmon is pricier but worth the splurge if it fits within your budget, since farm raised often contains pollutants. Mild, slightly sweet baby bok choy is loaded with nutrients, including vitamin C and folate, and it's super easy to prepare. Whisk together the quick, flavorful sauce and you're good to go in just a few minutes. Serve warm with steamed rice. Cover and refrigerate leftovers for up to two days.

4 teaspoons avocado or extra-virgin olive oil

3 tablespoons coconut aminos

1½ teaspoons unseasoned rice vinegar

4 teaspoons white miso

1½ teaspoons Dijon mustard

¼ teaspoon toasted sesame oil

1 teaspoon maple syrup

1 clove garlic, grated

½ teaspoon grated fresh ginger

1½ pounds salmon (preferably wild caught) cut into 4 equal portions, patted dry

4 heads baby bok choy, quartered

Kosher salt and freshly ground black pepper

2 teaspoons toasted sesame seeds

2 scallions (white and light green parts only), thinly sliced on a diagonal

RECIPE CONTINUES

1. Preheat the oven to 425°F. Line a baking sheet with parchment paper and drizzle with 2 teaspoons of avocado oil.

2. In a shallow dish, combine the coconut aminos, vinegar, miso, mustard, sesame oil, maple syrup, garlic, and ginger; whisk to mix well.

3. Place the salmon, skin side down, on the prepared baking sheet. Place the bok choy, cut side down, around the salmon. Drizzle the salmon and bok choy with the remaining avocado oil and season with a few pinches of salt and pepper.

4. Pour the coconut aminos mixture over the salmon and bok choy, making sure to coat evenly. Sprinkle the salmon with the sesame seeds. Bake until the salmon is cooked to the desired doneness (120°F for medium-rare, up to 145°F for fully cooked through), 12 to 15 minutes. Sprinkle the scallions over the salmon and serve.

NOTE

You'll find miso, a fermented paste usually made from soybeans, in the refrigerated section of your supermarket. It will keep in the fridge for a few months (press a sheet of plastic wrap directly onto the paste before covering it to keep it fresh). Use it in dressings, sauces, and soups—try adding a little to anything that needs a deeper flavor. The darker the miso, the saltier and more strongly flavored it is; I like a relatively mild white miso for this recipe.

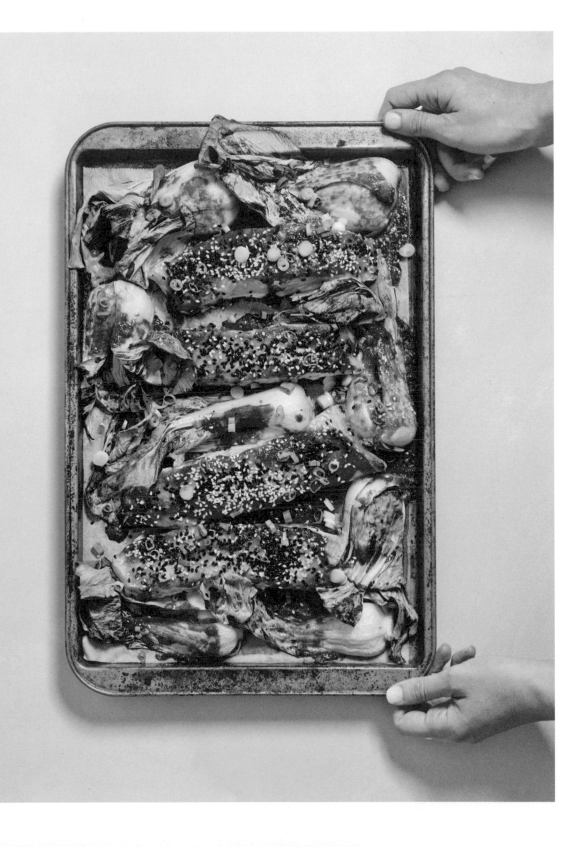

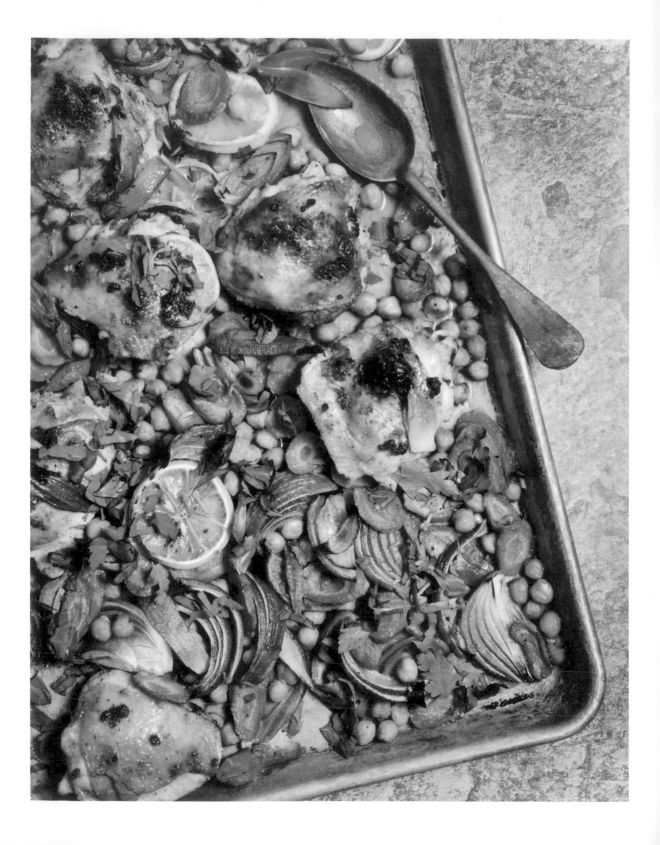

Chicken Thighs with Roasted Carrots, Onions, and Chickpeas

PREP TIME: 15 MINUTES | MARINATE TIME: 30 MINUTES | COOK TIME: 35 TO 40 MINUTES | YIELD: 4 SERVINGS

Boneless, skinless chicken breasts get all the love, but bone-in, skin-on thighs pack a lot of nutrition, have tons of flavor, and are budget-friendly too. Because they stay juicy even with a longer roasting time, you can cook them alongside the vegetables, so this dish is simple to throw together. Plan for at least thirty minutes of marinating time for the chicken, or up to six hours for even more luscious flavor.

1½ teaspoons onion powder

1½ teaspoons ground cumin

1 teaspoon ground coriander

4 garlic cloves, grated

4 teaspoons kosher salt

¼ teaspoon freshly ground black pepper

¼ teaspoon ground ginger

1 lemon, thinly sliced, seeds removed, plus extra lemon wedges for serving (optional)

5 tablespoons extra-virgin olive oil

8 bone-in, skin-on chicken thighs, trimmed of excess skin, patted dry

6 carrots, sliced ¼-inch thick on a diagonal

2 large red onions, thickly sliced

1 (14-ounce) can chickpeas, drained and rinsed

1 teaspoon garlic powder

¼ cup fresh, finely chopped flat-leaf parsley (optional)

1. Make the marinade: In a large bowl, combine the onion powder, cumin, coriander, garlic, 2 teaspoons of the salt, pepper, ginger, lemon slices, and 3 tablespoons of the oil. Place the chicken thighs in the bowl and toss to combine, rubbing the spices into the chicken. Cover and refrigerate for at least 30 minutes, or up to 6 hours.

RECIPE CONTINUES

2. Preheat the oven to 400°F. Line a baking sheet with a silicone mat. Spread the carrots, onions, and chickpeas onto the prepared baking sheet. Drizzle with the remaining 2 tablespoons of oil, garlic powder, the remaining 2 teaspoons of salt, and pepper to taste. Toss to combine and spread evenly into a single layer.

3. Tuck the chicken thighs between the vegetables and bake until the chicken is cooked through (an instant-read thermometer stuck into the thickest part away from the bone should read 170°F), 30 to 35 minutes.

4. Switch the oven to broil. Place the baking sheet on the middle rack, about 6 to 8 inches from the heat source. Broil on high until the chicken skin is golden brown and crispy, 3 to 5 minutes. Portion the chicken and vegetables onto four plates; season with additional salt and pepper, if needed. Sprinkle on the parsley and serve with the lemon wedges, if desired.

NOTES

Chickpeas are also called garbanzo beans, and you can find them in the canned foods aisle (or get dried ones, then soak them before cooking for a budget-friendly option that you can keep on hand).

The liquid on the baking sheet after roasting is super flavorful, so brush or drizzle it on the chicken and vegetables before sprinkling it with the parsley.

Lemon Sole with Fried Capers

PREP TIME: 15 MINUTES | COOK TIME: 10 MINUTES | YIELD: 4 SERVINGS

Imagine chicken piccata with mild white fish instead of chicken, and that's basically what you have here. It's loaded with flavor but on the table in under thirty minutes, perfect for busy weeknights. Lemon sole is mild and light, not fishy, so it's still appetizing in those moments when most seafood is a turnoff. Plus, it's budget-friendly and relatively low in mercury, so it's a go-to option in pregnancy. Be sure to pat it dry thoroughly before cooking.

1½ tablespoons fresh lemon juice

3 tablespoons low-sodium chicken bone broth or vegetable broth

½ teaspoon arrowroot flour

1½ tablespoons unsalted butter

1½ teaspoons extra-virgin olive oil

2 tablespoons drained capers, patted dry

1 pound lemon sole, cut into 4 pieces, thoroughly patted dry

½ teaspoon fine sea salt

¼ teaspoon freshly ground black pepper

½ teaspoon garlic powder

1. In a cup, combine the lemon juice and broth. Dissolve the arrowroot in half a teaspoon of water; stir into the broth mixture.

2. In a large nonstick skillet, melt the butter with the oil over medium heat. Add the capers and cook, stirring, until hot and lightly toasted, 2 to 3 minutes. Remove with a slotted spoon and transfer to a cup.

3. Season the fish all over with salt, pepper, and garlic powder. Add it to the hot skillet and cook until it's light golden on one side, 2 to 3 minutes.

RECIPE CONTINUES

Flip and cook until cooked through, 1 to 2 minutes longer. Divide among four plates.

4. Stir the lemon juice mixture and add it to the skillet. Cook, stirring, until warmed through and thickened, 30 to 60 seconds. Spoon evenly on top of the fish, sprinkle with the capers, and serve.

Chicken Egg Roll Bowl

PREP TIME: 20 MINUTES | COOK TIME: 20 MINUTES | YIELD: 4 SERVINGS

All the goodness of an egg roll minus the fried wrapping. Hearty and satisfying, this dish has tons of tastiness and loads of vegetables, and it comes together in a snap, thanks to the pre-shredded coleslaw mix. You can swap in a different protein here, such as shrimp or tofu. Make sure you have all the ingredients prepped before you turn on the stove; as with all stir-fries, once you start cooking, it moves fast.

1 teaspoon arrowroot flour or cornstarch

6 tablespoons coconut aminos

½ teaspoon raw honey

1½ teaspoons unseasoned rice vinegar (or cider vinegar)

1 teaspoon sriracha, plus more for serving (optional)

2 large eggs

2½ tablespoons avocado oil

¾ teaspoon fine sea salt

1 pound boneless, skinless chicken thighs, trimmed and cut into 1-inch pieces

4 scallions, white and light green parts only, sliced on a diagonal (about ⅓ cup); dark green parts sliced and reserved for garnish (optional)

1 cup snow peas, sliced on a diagonal

3 garlic cloves, minced

1 tablespoon grated fresh ginger

1 (12-ounce) bag coleslaw mix (shredded cabbage and carrots)

1 tablespoon toasted sesame oil, plus more to taste

Hoisin sauce, for serving (optional)

1. In a small cup, dissolve the arrowroot in 1 teaspoon of water. In a small bowl, whisk together 5 tablespoons of the coconut aminos, the honey, vinegar, and sriracha, if using. In a small bowl, beat the eggs with the remaining 1 tablespoon of coconut aminos.

RECIPE CONTINUES

2. In a medium skillet, warm $1/2$ tablespoon of the avocado oil over medium heat. Pour in the egg mixture, season with $1/8$ teaspoon of the salt, and cook, stirring constantly and breaking it into pieces as it firms up, until just cooked through, 2 to 3 minutes. Transfer to a medium bowl and cover.

3. In a large skillet, warm 1 tablespoon of the avocado oil over medium-high heat. Add the chicken, season with $1/4$ teaspoon of the salt, and cook, stirring, until cooked through, 5 to 7 minutes. Transfer to the bowl with the eggs; cover to keep warm. If there's excess liquid in the skillet, pour it off.

4. In the large skillet, warm the remaining 1 tablespoon of avocado oil. Add the white and light green scallions and snow peas; sprinkle with $1/8$ teaspoon of the salt and cook, stirring, for 1 minute. Add the garlic and ginger; stir-fry for 1 minute, until fragrant. Add the coleslaw mix; season with the remaining $1/4$ teaspoon of salt and stir-fry until tender, 2 to 3 minutes.

5. Reduce the heat to medium. Add the chicken and egg back to the skillet along with any juices that have collected in the bowl. Whisk the coconut aminos mixture and pour it into the skillet, stirring to pull up any browned bits from the bottom of the skillet. Drizzle in the arrowroot mixture and cook, stirring, until the sauce reduces and thickens and coats all the ingredients in the skillet, about 1 minute longer.

6. Remove from the heat and drizzle with the sesame oil. Season with additional salt and/or sesame oil, if needed. Serve, garnishing with the optional dark scallion greens. Pass sriracha and hoisin on the side, if using.

NOTE

You can make this dish with tofu instead of chicken. Skip step 3. Cut a block of baked tofu into cubes or strips and add it during the last minute of cooking the coleslaw mix. Stir carefully to keep it from breaking up.

Salmon Poke-Inspired Bowls

PREP TIME: 10 MINUTES | COOK TIME: 20 MINUTES | YIELD: 2 SERVINGS

Are you missing sushi? This poke-inspired bowl is a pregnancy-friendly substitute for the traditional raw version with all the familiar ingredients and tastes. The marinade and quick cooking method ensure the salmon is super delicious and super tender. Nori is the seaweed that is typically wrapped around sushi in restaurants. You can buy sheets of it, cut it into squares, and use it to wrap the filling ingredients to create little sushi bites.

SALMON

1 pound boneless, skinless salmon fillet, patted dry, cut into 1-inch chunks

1 teaspoon toasted sesame oil

2 tablespoons coconut aminos

1 teaspoon kosher salt

1 teaspoon ground ginger

½ teaspoon onion powder

1 tablespoon avocado oil

SUSHI RICE

1 cup short-grain rice

2 tablespoons unseasoned rice vinegar

1 teaspoon sugar

1½ teaspoons salt

BOWLS

1 ripe avocado, thinly sliced

1 large carrot, shredded

2 Persian cucumbers, diced into small cubes

RECIPE CONTINUES

2 scallions (white and light green parts only), thinly sliced

2 teaspoons toasted sesame seeds

2 large sheets toasted nori, cut into 4 squares

1. In a bowl, combine the salmon, sesame oil, coconut aminos, salt, ginger, and onion powder. Toss to combine. Cover and refrigerate while you prepare the rice and cut the vegetables.

2. While the salmon is marinating, cook the sushi rice according to the package directions. Once the rice is finished cooking, in a small saucepan, warm the vinegar, sugar, and salt until the sugar and salt dissolve. Spread the cooked rice out onto a baking sheet and evenly distribute the vinegar mixture over it. Use a small spatula to gently fold and fluff the rice; this will help to distribute the seasoning and create more starch to help the rice stick together. Remove the salmon from the marinade with a slotted spoon and discard any leftover marinade. In a large skillet, warm the avocado oil over medium-high heat. Add the salmon and cook, stirring occasionally, until hot and lightly browned, about 3 to 4 minutes.

3. Assemble the bowls: Divide the rice between two bowls. Arrange the salmon, avocado, carrot, and cucumbers over the top. Sprinkle with the scallions and sesame seeds, and serve with the nori squares.

NOTES

For a shortcut, use microwaveable organic rice. Remove it from the container, put it in a glass bowl with a microwave-safe cover, and cook according to the package directions.

You can ask your fishmonger to remove the salmon skin for you. But don't toss it—warm it in a skillet with a bit of oil and salt, turning it over a few times, until crisp and golden. Crumble it on top of your poke bowl.

Whisk sriracha and coconut aminos into a spoonful of mayo and drizzle it onto your bowl for extra spice.

MAKE-AHEAD MEALS

Bone Broth

PREP TIME: 10 MINUTES | COOK TIME: 12 TO 24 HOURS |
YIELD: 10 (1-CUP) SERVINGS

Bone broth is easy to make if you have a large slow cooker (though you can also make it on the stovetop; see Note). Freeze it in one-cup servings, or it will keep in the fridge for up to four days.

You can also save veggie peels and trimmings from onions, celery, carrots, and mushrooms, along with herb stems from fresh rosemary or thyme and peels from fresh garlic. Keep in a one-gallon zipper bag in the freezer, and then keep chicken bones and the carcass from a roasted chicken in another one-gallon zipper bag. When both are full, use them in place of the chicken backs or wings and veggies.

This recipe has no salt added so the broth can be added to soups and then seasoned to taste.

1 onion (peel and root still on), cut into quarters

2 carrots, roughly chopped

1 celery stalk, roughly chopped

4 garlic cloves (peel on), lightly smashed

2 tablespoons apple cider vinegar

10 peppercorns

2 pounds chicken wings or backs, skin removed

RECIPE CONTINUES

1. Place all ingredients in a slow cooker. Fill with water to half an inch below the rim. Cover and cook on low for 12 to 24 hours.

2. Strain through a fine mesh sieve and discard the solids.

NOTE

Stovetop instructions: Over medium-high heat, bring the bone broth to a simmer, uncovered. As soon as the bone broth begins to simmer, turn the heat down to the lowest setting. Allow to simmer for one hour, uncovered, skimming any foam that rises to the top. After an hour, cover the bone broth and cook on the lowest setting for 12 to 24 hours. Strain through a fine mesh sieve and discard the solids.

VARIATIONS

Add a 1-inch knob of ginger root, peeled and roughly chopped, and 1 star anise to make pho-inspired broth.

Sausage and Zucchini Lasagna

PREP TIME: 40 MINUTES | COOK TIME: 1 HOUR 30 MINUTES | YIELD: 6 TO 8 SERVINGS

If there's a dish as comforting and satisfying as lasagna, I haven't had it. No-boil noodles streamline the process, and the sausage and zucchini add heft and a touch of green to the dish. Use sweet or hot Italian sausage ("sweet" isn't actually sweet; it just means not spicy). If you use a glass baking dish with rounded edges, break off tiny corners of the noodles so they lay flat inside.

2 teaspoons avocado oil

10 ounces sweet or hot Italian sausage, casings removed (2 large links)

1 medium zucchini, ends trimmed, quartered lengthwise, and cut into ⅛-inch slices

⅛ plus ¼ teaspoon salt

2 large eggs

1 (15-ounce) container ricotta

4 cups shredded mozzarella

¾ cup freshly grated Parmesan

2 teaspoons Italian seasoning

Pinch of ground nutmeg

¼ teaspoon freshly ground black pepper

2 (24-ounce) jars marinara

1 (9-ounce) box no-boil lasagna noodles

Olive oil cooking spray

1. Preheat the oven to 375°F. In a large skillet, warm the oil over medium heat. Add the sausage and cook, stirring and breaking up the meat, until it is cooked through and lightly browned in spots, 7 to 10 minutes. Use a slotted spoon to transfer the sausage to a bowl, leaving any fat behind (if there's no fat, add another teaspoon or two of oil). Add the zucchini to the skillet; season with the ⅛ teaspoon of salt. Cook, stirring occasionally, until the zucchini is tender and lightly caramelized in

RECIPE CONTINUES

spots, 6 to 8 minutes. Transfer to the bowl with the sausage; stir to combine.

2. In a large bowl, beat the eggs. Add the ricotta, 2 cups of the mozzarella, $1/2$ cup of the Parmesan, Italian seasoning, nutmeg, the $1/4$ teaspoon of salt, and pepper.

3. Spread 1 cup of the marinara sauce into the bottom of a 9 × 13-inch baking dish. Add 4 noodles, overlapping slightly. Spread half the ricotta mixture on top, then sprinkle half the sausage mixture over evenly. Sprinkle with 1 cup of mozzarella. Spread $1^1/2$ cups of sauce over.

4. Top with another layer of 4 noodles, the remaining ricotta mixture, the remaining sausage mixture, and $1^1/2$ cups of sauce. Cover with 4 noodles, 1 cup of sauce, and the remaining 1 cup of mozzarella. Sprinkle with the remaining $1/4$ cup of Parmesan.

5. Mist one side of a large sheet of foil with cooking spray; cover the baking dish with the foil, spray side down. Bake for 50 to 60 minutes, until the noodles are tender and the lasagna is bubbly. Uncover and bake until the cheese on top has fully melted, 5 to 10 minutes longer. Let stand for at least 15 minutes before serving, or let cool, cover, and refrigerate.

NOTES

Place a sheet of foil that's larger than the baking dish under the dish to catch any drips.

You can use turkey sausage instead of pork.

Change up the sauce. An arrabbiata will make the lasagna spicier; a vodka sauce will make it creamier. Or use a sauce that includes vegetables, like mushrooms and/or onions.

Lasagna is even better the day after it's cooked. Let it cool completely, then cover and refrigerate. Cover to reheat the whole thing, or warm individual pieces. It also freezes well, either whole or in pieces. Thaw in the fridge overnight before rewarming.

Classic Meatballs

PREP TIME: 20 MINUTES | COOK TIME: 20 TO 25 MINUTES |
YIELD: 8 SERVINGS (7 TO 8 MEATBALLS EACH)

Meatballs are a versatile pre-made food you can store in your freezer. Use them in soups, add them to pasta sauce, serve them as appetizers, or enjoy them over regular noodles, cooked zucchini noodles, or spaghetti squash or simply reheat them and serve with a salad and a side. They're also super easy to adapt to a flavor profile, what you make them from, and more. This recipe uses two pounds of meat, which is about sixty 1½-inch meatballs. Since this recipe makes a lot, you can freeze some for later. I like to store them in single servings for those nights when I just need something quick.

½ cup milk of choice

½ cup dried bread crumbs (or gluten-free bread crumbs)

2 tablespoons extra-virgin olive oil

1 yellow onion, finely minced

2 carrots, grated

3 garlic cloves, minced

1 pound lean ground beef

1 pound ground pork or ground turkey breast

¼ cup freshly grated Parmesan (optional)

2 large eggs, lightly beaten

1 tablespoon dried thyme

1 teaspoon salt

¼ teaspoon freshly ground black pepper

1. Preheat the oven to 400°F. Line a rimmed baking sheet with parchment paper.

2. In a small bowl, mix the milk and bread crumbs. Mix until the bread completely absorbs the liquid. Set aside. This is called a panade, and mixing the milk and bread crumbs this way will help keep your meatballs soft and moist regardless of the type of ground meat you use.

RECIPE CONTINUES

3. In a large skillet, heat the oil on medium-high until it shimmers.

4. Add the onions and carrots. Cook, stirring occasionally, until the veggies are very soft, 3 to 4 minutes.

5. Add the garlic and cook, stirring constantly, for 30 seconds. Remove from the heat and let cool completely.

6. In a large bowl, combine the ground beef, ground pork, panade, cooled veggies, optional Parmesan, eggs, thyme, salt, and pepper. Mix well.

7. Form into 1½-inch meatballs. Place the meatballs onto the prepared baking sheet.

8. Bake until the meatballs reach an internal temperature of 165°F, about 20 minutes.

9. To freeze, cool completely before dividing into single-serving bags (7 to 8 meatballs) that are clearly labeled with the contents and the date. They'll keep for about 6 months. Reheat from frozen in a 350°F oven for about 20 minutes.

VARIATIONS

For Mediterranean-inspired meatballs: Replace the ground beef and ground pork with 2 pounds of ground lamb. Increase the garlic to 6 cloves. Replace the thyme with 1 teaspoon of dried oregano and ½ teaspoon of dried marjoram.
For poultry-based meatballs: Replace the ground beef and ground pork with 1 pound each of ground chicken and ground turkey (or 2 pounds of one or the other).

Simple Beef Stew

PREP TIME: 20 MINUTES | COOK TIME: 1½ TO 2 HOURS | YIELD: 4 TO 6 SERVINGS

Don't be scared by the long cooking time in this recipe; most of it is hands-off, with the stew lightly bubbling away in the oven. The stew meat is a tough cut, and the long, slow, low-temperature cooking makes it super tender. Pomegranate juice stands in for wine here—you'll love the complex flavor it lends to this rich dish. If you have leftovers, freeze them in single-serve containers for up to six months (perfect for a quick, hearty meal after the baby comes).

2½ pounds beef chuck, cut into 2-inch chunks, patted dry

3 teaspoons kosher salt

¾ teaspoon freshly ground black pepper

2 tablespoons avocado oil, plus more as needed

1 large yellow onion, chopped

3 celery stalks, chopped

4 carrots, sliced ½ inch thick on a diagonal

6 garlic cloves, minced (about 2 tablespoons)

1 cup unsweetened pomegranate juice

3 large Yukon Gold potatoes, cut into 1-inch chunks

1 large sprig fresh rosemary

2 dried bay leaves

4 cups low-sodium beef bone broth

1 cup frozen peas

4 teaspoons cornstarch or tapioca starch

¼ cup fresh flat-leaf parsley, roughly chopped

Thinly sliced chives for serving (optional)

1. Preheat the oven to 325°F. Toss the beef with 2 teaspoons of the salt and ½ teaspoon of the pepper.

RECIPE CONTINUES

2. In a large Dutch oven, warm the oil over medium-high heat. Working in batches, add the beef to the pot in a single layer. Sear the meat until browned on all sides, turning every 2 to 3 minutes with tongs (it will not be cooked through; that's okay). Transfer to a large bowl. Repeat for as many rounds as necessary without overcrowding the pot, adding more oil between batches, if needed.

3. If there's no fat left in the Dutch oven, add a few teaspoons of oil. Add the onions, celery, and carrots to the pot; season with the remaining 1 teaspoon of salt and the remaining 1/4 teaspoon of pepper. Cook, stirring occasionally, until the vegetables are tender, about 5 minutes. Add the garlic; sauté until fragrant, 30 seconds to 1 minute.

4. Pour in the pomegranate juice and cook, stirring with a wooden spoon to pull up the browned bits from the bottom of the pot. Cook, stirring occasionally, until the juice has reduced, 5 to 10 minutes. Add the potatoes, the beef and any juices that have collected in the bowl, rosemary, bay leaves, and beef bone broth. Bring to a boil, then cover and place in the oven. Cook until the beef is very tender and easily pulled apart with a fork, 1 hour 30 minutes to 2 hours.

5. Place the pot back on the stove over medium-low heat. Carefully remove the rosemary stem and bay leaves and stir in the frozen peas. In a small bowl, combine the cornstarch and 1 tablespoon of water, stirring until dissolved. Stir the cornstarch mixture into the stew and cook gently, stirring occasionally, until it thickens, about 1 minute. Ladle the stew into bowls, top with the parsley and chives, if using, and serve.

Lentil and Root Vegetable Stew

PREP TIME: 15 MINUTES | COOK TIME: 30 TO 40 MINUTES |
YIELD: 6 (2-CUP) SERVINGS

Lentils are inexpensive, versatile, and a good source of quick energy and protein. You can precook them and freeze in 1-cup portions in bags for up to six months, so you always have cooked lentils available.

This stew calls for precooked lentils. Cook raw lentils in water with a bay leaf using the package directions (boil for about 20 minutes or until tender, drain, cool, and refrigerate, freeze, or use).

2 tablespoons extra-virgin olive oil

1 yellow onion, chopped

4 garlic cloves, minced

1 tablespoon tomato paste

4 cups low-sodium vegetable broth

1 tablespoon Dijon mustard

2 sweet potatoes, peeled and cut into 1-inch cubes

2 celery stalks, chopped

2 large carrots (or three medium), chopped

2 medium turnips, peeled and chopped

1 bay leaf

1 teaspoon dried thyme

1 teaspoon fine sea salt

¼ teaspoon freshly ground black pepper

3 cups cooked lentils

2 tablespoons cornstarch or arrowroot flour

¼ cup red wine vinegar

1. In a large pot, heat the oil on medium-high until it shimmers.

2. Add the onions and cook, stirring occasionally, until soft, 5 to 7 minutes.

3. Add the garlic and cook, stirring constantly, for 30 seconds.

RECIPE CONTINUES

4. Add the tomato paste, broth, and mustard, whisking to combine. Bring to a boil.

5. Add the sweet potatoes, celery, carrots, turnips, bay leaf, thyme, salt, and pepper.

6. Bring to a boil. Reduce the heat to medium. Simmer, stirring occasionally, until the vegetables are tender, 20 to 25 minutes.

7. Add the lentils. Cook to heat through, 3 to 5 minutes more.

8. In a small bowl, whisk together the cornstarch and vinegar. Pour into the stew while stirring.

9. Continue to simmer until the stew thickens, about 2 more minutes. Remove and discard the bay leaf before serving or freezing.

SLOW COOKER INSTRUCTIONS

1. Omit the oil. In a slow cooker, combine the onions, garlic, tomato paste, broth, mustard, sweet potatoes, celery, carrots, turnips, bay leaf, thyme, salt, and pepper.
2. Cover and cook on low for 8 hours or on high for 4 hours.
3. Uncover. Stir in the lentils. While the lentils warm, whisk together the cornstarch and vinegar. Add to the uncovered slow cooker while stirring. Cook, stirring, just until the sauce thickens, about 5 minutes more.

NOTES

In place of the turnips, you could use 1 celery root, 2 to 3 parsnips, a fennel bulb, or even a potato.

If you want to add green leafy veggies like spinach or kale, add them at the end. They will heat quickly in the warm stew; just rest it for 5 minutes or so (even with the heat off) before serving. You can even do this in the slow cooker. Simply add the greens at the end of cooking and give the stew an additional 5 minutes.

LACTOGENIC RECIPES

Citrusy Beet and Barley Salad

PREP TIME: 25 MINUTES | COOK TIME: 45 MINUTES | YIELD: 4 TO 6 SERVINGS

This vibrant salad offers a satisfying combination of tastes and textures. Barley, aside from being hearty and yummy, is a lactogenic food, so this meal also supports your milk supply. The crunchy almonds, creamy goat cheese, and antioxidant-rich, earthy beets in it are all loaded with nutrients. Keep leftovers covered in the fridge and pick on them for up to four days. Note that eating beets can turn your pee or stool bright red—this is perfectly normal, so don't be alarmed.

CITRUS VINAIGRETTE

Juice of 1 medium orange (¼ cup)

Juice of ½ lemon (2 to 3 tablespoons)

1 teaspoon Dijon mustard

3 tablespoons extra-virgin olive oil

Kosher salt

Freshly ground black pepper

SALAD

2 pounds beets (about 4 large), yellow or red, scrubbed and patted dry

1½ tablespoons extra-virgin olive oil

1 teaspoon kosher salt, plus more to taste

1 cup pearl barley

RECIPE CONTINUES

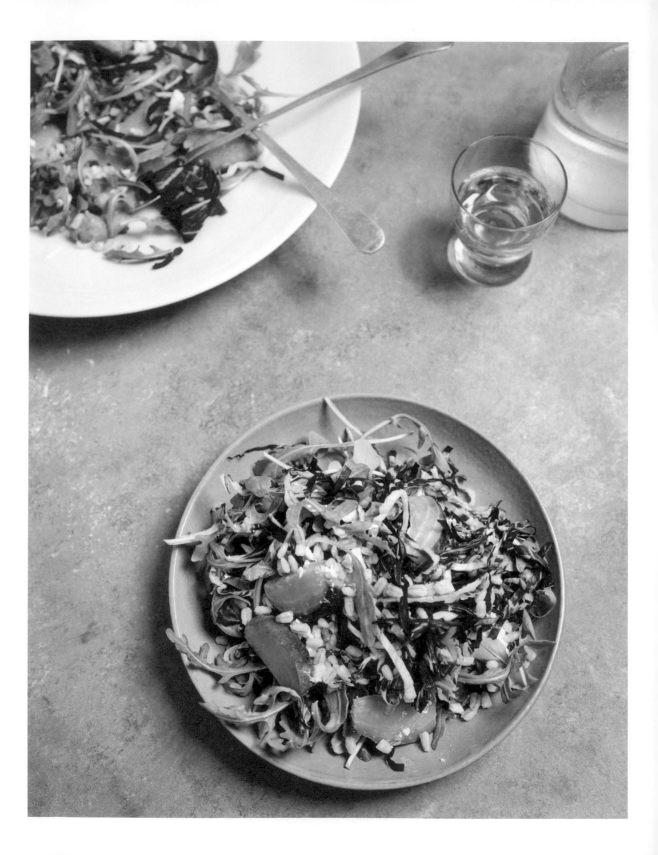

3 cups low-sodium chicken bone broth or water

1 cup arugula

1 large head radicchio, shredded

Freshly ground black pepper

½ cup raw whole almonds, roughly chopped

¾ cup crumbled feta

1. Make the vinaigrette: In a medium bowl, whisk together the orange and lemon juices and mustard. Whisking constantly, slowly drizzle in the oil until well mixed. Season with salt and pepper to taste. (Alternatively, put all the ingredients except the salt and pepper in a jar, cover, and shake vigorously to mix, then season with salt and pepper to taste.) You can make the vinaigrette up to a day ahead; cover and keep it at room temperature. Mix well before using.

2. Preheat the oven to 375°F. Line a large rimmed baking sheet with parchment paper.

3. Using a sharp chef's knife, slice off the roots and the tips of the beets. With a flat end on the cutting board, slice each beet in half. Place cut side down and slice the halves into ½-inch-thick wedges. Place the beets onto the prepared baking sheet; drizzle with the oil and sprinkle with the salt. Roast until the beets are easily pierced with a fork, 30 to 35 minutes. Let the beets cool on the baking sheet, then transfer them to a large bowl.

4. Meanwhile, prepare the barley. In a large saucepan, combine the barley, broth, and a pinch of salt. Bring to a boil over high heat, then reduce the heat to low and simmer uncovered until the barley is tender and most of the liquid has been absorbed, 25 to 30 minutes. Spread the barley onto a baking sheet to cool. (This will help it to cool faster; if you have more time, you can put it in a large bowl and stir it occasionally.) Add the cooled barley to the bowl with the beets.

RECIPE CONTINUES

5. Add the arugula and radicchio to the bowl. Add the vinaigrette and toss to coat, adding 1 tablespoon at a time, tossing to coat until the salad is dressed to your liking. Season with salt and pepper to taste. Top with the almonds and feta and serve.

NOTE

You can change up this salad so it suits your taste and what you have on hand. Swap soft goat cheese or shredded ricotta salata for the feta, or toss in chopped toasted pistachios for the almonds.

Energy Bites

Energy Bites are an easy-to-make, endlessly variable, sweet, and chewy snack that is also full of good-for-you ingredients. These are made with dried dates, which have fiber and minerals and may ease labor and delivery, and a caramellike taste that can really help with those sweet cravings. One version has bright lemon and rich coconut, and the other has lactogenic oats and will remind you of an oatmeal-chocolate-chip cookie. Keep them in the fridge to grab and go, or make a double batch and freeze some for future snack emergencies.

LEMON-COCONUT ENERGY BITES

PREP TIME: 15 MINUTES | YIELD: ABOUT 32 ENERGY BITES

$1/2$ cup almonds (raw or roasted)

$1/2$ cup raw cashews

Generous pinch of fine sea salt

2 cups pitted dates

2 teaspoons grated lemon zest

$1/4$ cup fresh lemon juice

$1/2$ cup unsweetened shredded coconut, plus more for rolling (optional)

2 tablespoons chia seeds

1. In a food processor, place the nuts and salt; pulse to chop. (Do not overprocess and turn the nuts into butter.) Transfer to a bowl.

2. Add the dates, zest, and juice to the processor; pulse to form a paste, stopping to scrape down the processor once or twice. Add the coconut and chia seeds; pulse several times until all the ingredients are well chopped and combined.

RECIPE CONTINUES

3. Use two spoons or a small ice-cream scoop to portion into balls. Roll in additional coconut, if desired. Store covered in the fridge for up to a week or in the freezer for up to two months.

OAT AND FLAX ENERGY BITES

PREP TIME: 15 MINUTES | YIELD: ABOUT 12 ENERGY BITES

$1^1/_2$ cup rolled oats
$^1/_2$ cup ground flaxseed
$^1/_4$ cup pure maple syrup or honey
$^1/_2$ cup creamy natural peanut butter or another nut or seed butter
1 teaspoon vanilla
$^3/_4$ cup chocolate chips
$^1/_2$ cup unsweetened coconut flakes

1. In a large bowl, mix together the oats, flaxseed, syrup or honey, peanut butter, and vanilla.

2. Fold in the chocolate chips.

3. Form into 1-inch balls and roll in the coconut flakes.

VARIATIONS

Roll the balls in slivered almonds or chopped pecans or walnuts.
Add dried fruit, such as dried apples, cranberries, or apricots, in place of the chocolate chips.
Add 1 tablespoon of chia seeds or flaxseeds to the dough.
Soak the dates in hot orange juice for citrus flavor.

PB&J Lactogenic Smoothie

PREP TIME: 5 MINUTES | YIELD: 1 SERVING

This smoothie is packed with science-backed ingredients to boost your milk supply, such as oats, nut butter, and brewer's yeast. Plus, it hits all the notes of a classic PB&J, so you'll look forward to enjoying it as a breakfast or snack. Brewer's yeast is a bit bitter, but the creamy deliciousness of the nut butter rounds it out. Double the recipe and freeze some in ice-pop molds for a fast and fun treat.

1 cup milk of choice

1 banana

⅓ cup rolled oats

1 cup frozen blueberries or blackberries

2 tablespoons peanut butter or other nut butter of choice

1 tablespoon brewer's yeast (preferably debittered)

Pinch of kosher salt

In a high-speed blender, combine all the ingredients and blend until smooth and creamy.

Chocolate Chip Lactation Cookies

PREP TIME: 15 MINUTES | COOK TIME: 10 MINUTES | YIELD: 16 TO 20 COOKIES

Who doesn't love a warm chocolate chip cookie? These gluten-free and refined sugar–free ones offer a milk-boosting bonus. Oat flour, oats, and brewer's yeast offer supportive nutrition—but the chocolate chips and cinnamon make it taste like a pure treat. Plus, the dough comes together quickly in a bowl, so no need to pull out the electric mixer. Pro tip: make these as a postpartum gift for a friend, or bring a batch to your new-moms group.

3 large eggs

1 cup coconut sugar

5 tablespoons (2.5 ounces) unsalted butter; melted and cooled

1 teaspoon vanilla extract

2 cups oat flour

¾ cup rolled oats

¼ cup brewer's yeast (preferably debittered)

½ teaspoon baking soda

½ teaspoon ground cinnamon

¼ teaspoon salt

⅔ cup dark chocolate chips

1. Preheat the oven to 350°F. Line two baking sheets with parchment paper.

2. In a large bowl, whisk the eggs, sugar, butter, and vanilla. In a separate bowl, whisk together the oat flour, oats, brewer's yeast, baking soda, cinnamon, and salt. Add the oat flour mixture to the egg mixture and mix until all the ingredients are well combined. Fold in the chocolate chips.

3. Using two tablespoons or a small ice cream scoop, portion the dough into 1½-tablespoon balls. Place them onto the prepared baking sheets, spacing them at least 2 inches apart. Bake 10 to 12 minutes, turning the baking sheets around and switching top to bottom halfway through.

4. Let the cookies cool on the baking sheets on cooling racks for 5 minutes, then transfer the cookies to the racks to cool completely.

NOTE

Oats are naturally gluten-free, but they're often grown near wheat fields, and cross contamination can occur. If you have celiac disease or a gluten sensitivity, be sure to buy certified gluten-free oats and oat flour.

Apple and Pear Baked Oatmeal

PREP TIME: 15 MINUTES | COOK TIME: 30 MINUTES | YIELD: 6 SERVINGS

This baked oatmeal is the ideal make-ahead breakfast; picture rolling out of bed and simply warming up a square. Dreamy! It includes warm cinnamon, sweet pears, and crunchy almonds, but feel free to experiment with other fruits, nuts, and spices. This oatmeal can be a blank canvas for whatever you have on hand or are craving. It cuts into mess-free squares, so you can take your breakfast on the go in a mason jar or glass container. Drizzle on nut or seed butter for extra protein.

2¾ cups rolled oats

2 teaspoons ground cinnamon

1 teaspoon baking powder

1 teaspoon kosher salt

½ cup maple syrup or raw honey

½ cup unsweetened applesauce

2 large eggs

1¼ cups milk of choice

¼ cup melted unsalted butter or coconut oil

1 cup chopped pears (add more if you like)

⅓ cup sliced almonds or nut of choice

1. Preheat the oven to 375°F. Grease an 8 × 8-inch baking dish.

2. In a large bowl combine oats, cinnamon, baking powder, and salt. In a separate bowl, combine maple syrup, applesauce, eggs, milk, and melted butter and whisk together.

3. Add the wet ingredients into the bowl with the oats and stir to combine. Fold in the pears and nuts and pour into the greased baking dish. Place in the middle of the oven and bake for 30 minutes.

4. Let cool completely before slicing. Wrap the squares individually and store in the fridge.

SWEETS

Chocolate Freezer Fudge Bites

PREP TIME: 15 MINUTES | FREEZE TIME: 1 HOUR | YIELD: APPROXIMATELY 16 PIECES, DEPENDING ON THE SIZE OF YOUR ICE CUBE TRAY

Freezer fudge is a lifesaver when you need a quick snack that is also rich and luscious. Though it feels like a treat, it also has plenty of healthy fats and fiber to keep you satisfied. This is a flexible recipe that you can change up based on what you have on hand; swap the nut butter, add a splash of vanilla or a sprinkle of toasted coconut—don't be afraid to experiment and make it your own.

1 cup coconut butter

⅓ cup almond butter, or other nut butter of choice

¼ cup unsweetened cacao or cocoa powder

Flaky sea salt, such as Maldon (optional)

1. In a small saucepan, melt the coconut butter over low heat, stirring often (watch it carefully so it doesn't scorch).

2. Meanwhile, in a medium bowl, combine the almond butter and cacao. Pour in the melted coconut butter and stir until well combined. Divide the mixture among the wells of an ice cube tray. Sprinkle each cube lightly with sea salt, if using. Freeze until firm, at least 1 hour.

3. Transfer the cubes to a large silicone or zipper bag and keep them frozen until ready to enjoy.

RECIPE CONTINUES

NOTES

Use any nut butter you like, and both smooth and crunchy will work. Tahini, a paste made from sesame seeds, also works well. If the coconut butter and nut butter are both unsweetened, you can add a tablespoon or two of maple syrup or honey to the fudge.

Keep the fudge frozen, as it will melt at room temperature. You can let it stand on the counter for a minute or two if it's too hard right out of the freezer. If you don't have a spare ice cube tray, you can make the fudge in a mini muffin tin lined with paper liners.

Avocado Chocolate Mousse

PREP TIME: 10 MINUTES | YIELD: 4 (1-CUP) SERVINGS

Sometimes you just need chocolate—and when you do, nothing satisfies like smooth, ultrarich mousse. This version uses avocado as the base instead of heavy cream and raw egg whites, so it's safer to consume and also sneaks in lots of good nutrition and fiber (don't worry, you won't taste the avocado).

2 medium ripe avocados

⅓ cup unsweetened cacao or cocoa powder

3 tablespoons maple syrup

¼ cup milk of choice

½ teaspoon vanilla extract

Pinch of fine sea salt or kosher salt

In a food processor or blender, combine all the ingredients and process until smooth, stopping to scrape down the bowl as needed. If the mousse is too thick, add more milk 1 or 2 teaspoons at a time and blend until it reaches the desired consistency. Serve, or wrap well and refrigerate for up to 2 days.

VARIATIONS

Add 1 teaspoon of grated orange zest for an orange-chocolate mousse.
Add 1 tablespoon of peanut butter for a peanut butter chocolate mousse. You'll likely need to add a few extra tablespoons of milk to adjust the texture.
Serve sprinkled with chopped walnuts, pecans, or toasted coconut flakes.
Top with fresh berries.

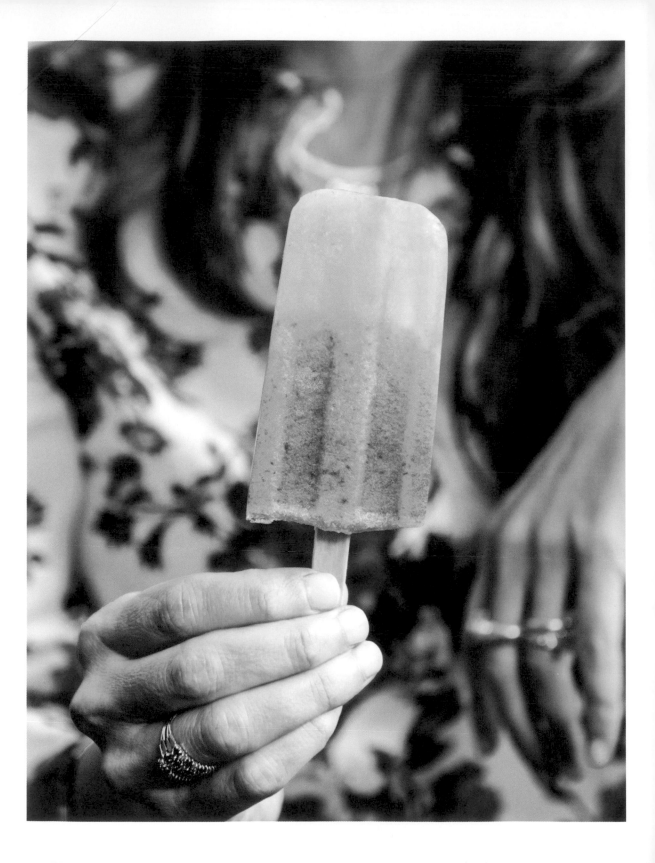

Mojito Ice Pops

PREP TIME: 15 MINUTES | FREEZE TIME: 4 HOURS | YIELD: ABOUT 2½ CUPS (5 POPS)

Here's the most fun way ever to get in your hydration. These ice pops have the sweet flavor of a mojito, with lime and mint (and they won't leave you with a hangover or sugar crash). They are cool and refreshing, since the cucumber base is 95 percent water, for a fabulous grown-up dessert or an after-workout cooldown treat.

1 medium English cucumber, chopped

Grated zest of 1 lime (about 1 tablespoon)

⅓ cup fresh lime juice

¼ cup raw honey

¼ cup fresh mint leaves

¼ teaspoon fine sea salt

In a blender, combine all the ingredients and blend until smooth. Divide the mixture among 5 (4-ounce) ice pop molds, insert the sticks, and freeze until firm, at least 4 hours, or overnight.

NOTES

You may need another tablespoon of honey, depending on how sweet your cucumber is. Taste the mixture after blending and add another 1 teaspoon at a time, if needed, to get to the sweetness you like.

Use just half of the cucumber and 1 cup of chopped seedless watermelon for a different taste.

Piña Colada Ice Pops

PREP TIME: 15 MINUTES | FREEZE TIME: 4 HOURS |
YIELD: ABOUT 2³/₄ CUPS (6 POPS)

Take a trip to the tropics right in your own kitchen by whipping up a batch of these pineapple-y, coconutty ice pops. They're fruity and refreshing. Don't skip the lime zest; it adds just a hint of complexity. And if you want to add another layer, sprinkle in a bit of chili powder or Tajín (a lime-chili seasoning I love).

1 (13.5-ounce) can full-fat coconut milk

1½ cups diced fresh pineapple

3 tablespoons maple syrup

1 teaspoon grated lime zest

1 teaspoon vanilla extract

¼ teaspoon fine sea salt

1. In a blender, combine all the ingredients. Blend until smooth.

2. Divide the mixture among 6 ice pop molds, add the sticks, and freeze until firm, at least 4 hours, or overnight.

NOTES

Fresh pineapple is best, diced finely. Canned diced pineapple doesn't have enough sweetness or flavor to hold its own. That being said, if fresh pineapple isn't available, use frozen or canned. Be sure the canned is packed in 100 percent juice, and pat off excess juice with a paper towel before using.

To up the coconut flavor, add ½ to 1 teaspoon of coconut extract.

Super-Fudgy Ice Pops

PREP TIME: 15 MINUTES | FREEZE TIME: 4 HOURS | YIELD: ABOUT 2 CUPS (5 POPS)

Enjoy what feels like an indulgence, knowing it's high in protein, low in sugar, and made with just a few wholesome ingredients. Thanks to a combo of cocoa and some melted chocolate chips, these pops are seriously fudgy and luscious.

½ cup chocolate chips

1 teaspoon unsalted butter or neutral oil (such as avocado)

1 cup plain Greek yogurt

½ cup milk of choice

3 tablespoons unsweetened cacao or cocoa powder

3 tablespoons maple syrup

1 teaspoon vanilla extract

Pinch of fine sea salt

1. In a small bowl, place the chocolate chips and butter. Set the bowl over a pan of simmering water and cook, stirring, until the chocolate is melted and smooth. Remove the bowl from the heat and let the mixture cool.

2. In a blender, combine the yogurt, milk, cacao or cocoa powder, maple syrup, vanilla, and salt; blend until combined. Add the chocolate mixture; blend again until smooth.

3. Divide the mixture among 5 ice pop molds, add the sticks, and freeze until firm, at least 4 hours, or overnight.

RESOURCES AND RECOMMENDED READING

Here are some of my favorite organizations and books, to help you throughout your pregnancy and postpartum.

CHAPTER ONE

- Third-party testing
  - NSF: Originally named the National Sanitation Foundation, NSF is an independent global organization founded in 1944 that facilitates public health standards and conducts and regulates product testing. An NSF certification guarantees top-notch third-party testing. nsf.org
  - Clean Label Project: A nonprofit dedicated to demystifying food labels and providing rigorous third-party testing for products. cleanlabelproject.org
  - Environmental Working Group (EWG): A nonprofit that educates consumers about products and practices that may be harmful to individuals or the environment. ewg.org

CHAPTER THREE

- Food safety: The FDA's at-a-glance list of food safety recommendations for pregnant women is an easy resource for knowing what to eat and what not to eat during pregnancy. In this book I've tried to provide a bit more nuance, but the FDA's recommendations are comprehensive. In addition, it provides excellent food handling and cleaning guidelines. fda.gov/food/people-risk-foodborne-illness/food-safety-mom-be-glance

- Foodborne illnesses: The FDA's chart of foodborne illnesses—including how they originate and how long they last—is an easy-to-follow guide. fda.gov/media/77727/download

- Fish and pregnancy
    - Environmental Defense Fund (EDF) Seafood Selector: The EDF's website includes information about mercury, environmental concerns, and recommended servings per month for various species of fish. seafood.edf.org
    - Monterey Bay Aquarium's Seafood Watch Guide: Available as a handy printable wallet card or searchable online database. seafoodwatch.org /globalassets/sfw/pdf/guides/seafood-watch-national-guide.pdf
    - Marine Stewardship Council (MSC): Here you can learn more about sustainable fishing and what the MSC's label and certification means on the seafood you buy. msc.org
    - Aquaculture Stewardship Council (ASC): Use the product locator (set the country filter to "United States" or other desired country) to get a list of certified seafood brands and products. us.asc-aqua.org

CHAPTER FOUR

- Toxins and pregnancy
    - The CDC provides a comprehensive list of toxic environmental exposures to avoid during pregnancy and postpartum. cdc.gov/niosh/topics/repro /specificexposures.html
    - I love the EWG's guide to green, healthy cleaning. It's long but worth a read! ewg.org/guides/cleaners/content/cleaners_and_health
    - The Campaign for Safe Cosmetics (CSC) is a great resource for finding safe, nontoxic beauty and personal-care products: safecosmetics.org

CHAPTER SIX

- Pregnancy and weight gain: The CDC and the American College of Obstetricians and Gynecologists (ACOG) have weight-gain charts based on BMI. Again, I don't recommend following these to a T, because every woman's body is different. cdc.gov/reproductivehealth /maternalinfanthealth/pregnancy-weight-gain.htm; acog.org/clinical /clinical-guidance/committee-opinion/articles/2013/01/weight-gain -during-pregnancy

- Gestational diabetes: I highly recommend *Real Food for Gestational Diabetes* by Lily Nichols, RDN, CDE, CLT. It is an invaluable and reassuring resource!

CHAPTER EIGHT

- Freezing food: I love this list of how long you can safely freeze foods. Thank you, FDA! fda.gov/media/74435/download

CHAPTER TEN

- Breastfeeding support: La Leche League International has been going strong since 1956, when a group of mothers realized they had no support (in a time when breastfeeding was often frowned upon), and it has provided invaluable assistance to women in the more than sixty years since. llli.org

- Breast milk testing: The Lactation Lab provides education and resources for nursing mothers, as well as testing breast milk for its nutritional content. lactationlab.com

- Milk banks: The Human Milk Banking Association of North America has a list of milk banks near you, as well as information on how you can donate or get the milk your baby needs. hmbana.org

ACKNOWLEDGMENTS

Just like a happy pregnancy, this book was both a labor of love and a true team effort. I am beyond lucky to have the support and participation of a team of all-stars, much like I did with *my* two pregnancies!

First, to my husband, Andrew. This book would not be possible without you. You saw it before I did. You are my idea person, a true collaborator and endless supporter. Thank you for your thoughtfulness, your ideas, your creativity, and your endless pep talks. Thank you for building me up when I didn't think I could do it and for keeping me on task. Most important, thank you for finding my literary agent, Kirsten Neuhaus!

Kirsten, thank you for your hands-on approach and collaboration. It is because of you that this book went from an idea to something real. You got it immediately and were a true champion. To my collaborator, Sarah Durand, thank you for being my constant sounding board, for your commitment and patience, and for answering my texts and emails at all hours—at and past deadlines. Honestly, this would still be a lot of words in numerous documents without you.

Thank you to the incredible talent who helped bring this to life. Beth Lipton, my constant collaborator and go-to for anything kitchen related. Amber Sauffer and Karen Frazier, you helped turn ideas into delicious reality. Rachel Kelly and Sarah Kamely, your additional expert eyes and fantastic research made sure I didn't miss a thing. To my Middleberg Nutrition team, Ayelet Schieber and Morgana Russino, thank you for your constant support through the years. And to Dr. Meredith Shur, thank you for taking the time to listen and answer my gazillion questions. It was beyond helpful.

To the amazing female-powerhouse creative team who brought life to these words: Photographer Gabriela Herman, who made it all look easy, vibrant, and beautiful. Food stylist Monica Pierini—I mean, while the food tastes great, you made it look even better! I also really appreciate your guidance through-out the entire process. And prop stylist Maeve Sheridan, you knew what I wanted to do even before I said it.

Thank you to my editor, Nina Shield; publisher, Megan Newman; associate editor, Hannah Steigmeyer; design director, Lorie Pagnozzi; and the entire Avery team: you believed in this book from the first pitch (at least I hope so!) and made the entire process so easy.

To my parents—my biggest supporters from day one—thanks for believing in me when I took the leap into the world of nutrition decades ago and for being constant listeners, therapists, business advisors, and everything else ever since. I also want to thank my wonderful sister and brother-in-law, Melissa and Jason Lupow, as well as my "I feel like I won the lottery" in-laws, Linda and Terry Kalish.

And last, to all my clients through the years. You are the inspiration for this book. Thank you for sharing your stories, your fears and worries, your successes, and most important, your beautiful children! Thank you for trusting me with yourselves and your families. You will see yourselves on each page.

NOTES

Chapter 2: Tests, Supplements, and Your First Trimester Nutritional Needs

23 **vegetarian pregnant women:** Roman Pawlak et al., "How Prevalent Is Vitamin B(12) Deficiency among Vegetarians?" *Nutrition Reviews* 71, no. 2 (February 2013): 110–17, doi.org/10.1111/nure.12001.

23 **B$_{12}$ deficient at delivery:** Carly E. Visentin et al., "Low Serum Vitamin B-12 Concentrations Are Prevalent in a Cohort of Pregnant Canadian Women," *The Journal of Nutrition* 146, no. 5 (May 2016): 1035–42, doi.org/10.3945/jn.115.226845.

24 **women who go off the pill:** Quaker E. Harmon, David M. Umbach, and Donna D. Baird, "Use of Estrogen-Containing Contraception Is Associated with Increased Concentrations of 25-Hydroxy Vitamin D," *The Journal of Clinical Endocrinology & Metabolism* 101, no. 9 (September 2016): 3370–77, doi.org/10.1210/jc.2016-1658.

25 **high hemoglobin A1c:** Otito Anaka et al., "Does First-Trimester Hemoglobin A1C Predict Gestational Diabetes and Fetal Outcome?" *Obstetrics & Gynecology* 123 (May 2014): 38S–39S, doi.org/10.1097/01.AOG.0000447315.90086.64.

27 **pregnant women are deficient:** Oladapo A. Ladipo, "Nutrition in Pregnancy: Mineral and Vitamin Supplements," *The American Journal of Clinical Nutrition* 72, no. 1 (July 2000): 280S–90S, doi.org/10.1093/ajcn/72.1.280S. PMID: 10871594; Sajin Bae et al., "Vitamin B-12 Status Differs among Pregnant, Lactating, and Control Women with Equivalent Nutrient Intakes," *The Journal of Nutrition* 146, no. 7 (July 2015): 1507–14, doi.org/10.3945/jn.115.210757; Lisa M. Bodnar et al., "High Prevalence of Vitamin D Insufficiency in Black and White Pregnant Women Residing in the Northern United States and Their Neonates," *The Journal of Nutrition* 137, no. 2 (February 2007): 447–52, doi.org/10.1093/jn/137.2.447.

34 **take 30 mg of iron a day:** "Iron: Fact Sheet for Health Professionals," Centers for Disease Control and Prevention, updated April 5, 2022, https://ods.od.nih.gov/factsheets/Iron-Consumer.

37 **attention spans of children:** Charlotte L. Bahnfleth et al., "Prenatal Choline Supplementation Improves Child Sustained Attention: A 7-year Follow-Up of a Randomized Controlled Feeding Trial," *The FASEB Journal* 36, no. 1 (January 2022): e22054, doi.org/10.1096/fj.202101217R.

38 **Vitamin D is a superstar:** Sina Gallo et al., "Vitamin D Supplementation during Pregnancy: An Evidence Analysis Center Systematic Review and Meta-Analysis," *Journal of the Academy of Nutrition and Dietetics* 120, no. 5 (October 25, 2019): 898–924.E4, doi.org/10.1016/j.jand.2019.07.002.

38 **Some studies even recommend four thousand:** Ambrish Mithal and Sanjay Kalra, "Vitamin D Supplementation in Pregnancy," *Indian Journal of Endocrinology and Metabolism* 18, no. 5 (September–October 2014): 593–96, doi.org/10.4103/2230-8210.139204.

39 **the inclusion of probiotic-rich foods:** Randi J. Bertelsen et al., "Probiotic Milk Consumption in Pregnancy and Infancy and Subsequent Childhood Allergic Diseases," *The Journal of Allergy and Clinical Immunology* 133, no. 1 (January 2014): 165–71.E8, doi.org/10.1016/j.jaci.2013.07.032; Samuli Rautava, Marko Kalliomäki, and Erika Isolauri, "Probiotics During Pregnancy and Breast-Feeding Might Confer Immunomodulatory Protection against Atopic Disease in the Infant" *The Journal of Allergy and Clinical Immunology* 109, no. 1 (January 2002): 119–21, doi.org/10.1067/mai.2002.120273.

39 **Magnesium deserves a special callout:** Joseph Cotruvo and Jamie Bartram, eds., "*Calcium and Magnesium in Drinking-water: Public Health Significance*," World Health Organization, 2009, who.int/publications/i/item/9789241563550.

41 **deficient in iodine:** Marica Krajcovicová-Kudláčková et al., "Iodine Deficiency in Vegetarians and Vegans," *Annals of Nutrition and Metabolism* 47, no. 5 (September–October 2003): 183–85, doi.org/10.1159/000070483.

41 **low levels of EPA and DHA:** Angela V. Saunders, Brenda C. Davis, and Manohar L. Garg, "Omega-3 Polyunsaturated Fatty Acids and Vegetarian Diets" *The Medical Journal of Australia* 199, no. S4 (June 2013): S22–S26, doi.org/10.5694/mja11.11507.

42 **Cast-iron skillets:** H. C. Brittin and C. E. Nossaman, "Iron Content of Food Cooked in Iron Utensils," *Journal of the American Dietetic Association* 86, no. 7 (July 1986): 897–901, PMID: 3722654.

Chapter 3: Foods to Nourish and Protect Mom

45 **your protein needs increase:** Rajavel Elango and Ronald O. Ball, "Protein and Amino Acid Requirements during Pregnancy," *Advances in Nutrition* 7, no. 4 (July 2016): 839S–44S, doi.org/10.3945/an.115.011817.

58 **Grass-fed livestock:** Cynthia A. Daley et al., "A Review of Fatty Acid Profiles and Antioxidant Content in Grass-Fed and Grain-Fed Beef," *Nutrition Journal* 9, no. 10 (March 10, 2010), doi.org/10.1186/1475-2891-9-10.

58 **48 percent less cadmium:** Marcin Barański, et al., "Higher Antioxidant and Lower Cadmium Concentrations and Lower Incidence of Pesticide Residues in Organically Grown Crops: A Systematic Literature Review and Meta-Analyses," *British Journal of Nutrition* 112, no. 5 (July 15, 2014): 794–811, doi.org/10.1017/S0007114514001366.

58 **preeclampsia and gestational diabetes:** Ebba Malmqvist et al., "Gestational Diabetes and Preeclampsia in Association with Air Pollution at Levels below Current Air Quality Guidelines,".*Environmental Health Perspectives* 121, no. 4 (April 1, 2013): 488–93, doi.org/10.1289/ehp.1205736.

58 **found in umbilical cord blood:** Jane Houlihan, et al., "Body Burden: The Pollution in Newborns," Environmental Working Group, July 14, 2005, https://www.ewg.org/research/body-burden-pollution-newborns.

73 **immune response is *stronger*:** Nima Aghaeepour et al., "An Immune Clock of Human Pregnancy," *Science Immunology* 2, no. 15 (September 1, 2017): eaan2946, doi/10.1126/sciimmunol.aan2946.

74 **seventeen times more likely:** Frederick S. Southwick and Daniel L. Purich, "Intracellular Pathogenesis of Listeriosis," *New England Journal of Medicine* 334, no. 12 (April 1996): 770–76, doi.org/10.1056/NEJM199603213341206.

74 **pasteurized cheese is considered safe:** Carolyn Tam, Aida Erebara, and Adrienne Einarson, "Food-Borne Illnesses during Pregnancy: Prevention and Treatment," *Canadian Family Physician* 56, no. 4 (April 2010): 341–43, PMID: 20393091.

76 **high levels of mercury exposure:** Pál Weihe et al., "Health Implications for Faroe Islanders of Heavy Metals and PCBs from Pilot Whales," *Science of the Total Environment* 186, no. 1–2 (July 16, 1996): 141–48, doi.org/10.1016/0048-9697(96)05094-2.

CHAPTER 4: NOURISHING AND PROTECTING BABY

88 **5.8 percent of children:** Benjamin Zablotsky, Lindsey I. Black, and Lara J. Akinbami, "Diagnosed Allergic Conditions in Children Aged 0–17 Years: United States, 2021," *NCHS Data Brief* 459 (January 2023), https://stacks.cdc.gov/view/cdc/123250.

88 **developing immune system:** Elisa Zubeldia-Varela et al., "Microbiome and Allergy: New Insights and Perspectives," *Journal of Investigational Allergology and Clinical Immunology* 32, no. 5 (2022): 327–44, doi.org/10.18176/jiaci.0852.

92 **lead and cadmium in cacao:** Eileen Abt et al., "Cadmium and Lead in Cocoa Powder and Chocolate Products in the US Market," *Food Additives & Contaminants: Part B, Surveillance* 11, no. 2 (June 2018): 92–102, doi.org/10.1080/19393210.2017.1420700.

95 **one out of twenty-four women:** "Exposures Add Up—Survey Results," Environmental Working Group, December 15, 2004, https://www.ewg.org/news-insights/news/2004/12/exposures-add-survey-results.

CHAPTER 6: FOOD-RELATED COMPLAINTS AND SIDE EFFECTS

123 **healthy weight range during pregnancy:** S. Lamina and E. Agbanusi, "Effect of Aerobic Exercise Training on Maternal Weight Gain in Pregnancy: A Meta-Analysis of Randomized Controlled Trials," *Ethiopian Journal of Health Sciences* 23, no. 1 (March 2013): 59–64, PMID: 23559839.

123 **help your body recover faster after:** Bradley B. Price, Saeid B. Amini, and Kaelyn Kappeler, "Exercise in Pregnancy: Effect on Fitness and Obstetric Outcomes—A Randomized Trial," *Medicine & Science in Sports & Exercise* 44, no. 12 (December 2012): 2263–69, doi.org/10.1249/MSS.0b013e318267ad67.

126 **unsweetened cranberry juice can reduce:** Jia-yue Xia et al., "Consumption of Cranberry as Adjuvant Therapy for Urinary Tract Infections in Susceptible Populations: A Systematic Review and Meta-Analysis with Trial Sequential Analysis," *PLoS One* 16, no. 9 (September 2, 2021): e0256992, doi.org/10.1371/journal.pone.0256992.

126 **"sticking" to the urinary tract wall:** Maryam Ghane, Laleh Babaeekhou, and Seyedeh Sepideh Ketabi, "Antibiofilm Activity of Kefir Probiotic Lactobacilli against Uropathogenic *Escherichia coli* (UPEC)," *Avicenna Journal of Medical Biotechnology* 12, no. 4 (October–December 2020): 221–29, PMID: 33014313.

128 **mental challenges, including anxiety:** M. Bicikova et al., "Vitamin D in Anxiety and Affective Disorders," *Physiological Research* 64, no. Suppl. 2 (2015): S101–3, doi.org/10.33549/physiolres.933082.

128 **Foods rich in zinc:** Mozhgan Torabi et al., "Effects of Nano and Conventional Zinc Oxide on Anxiety-Like Behavior in Male Rats," *Indian Journal of Pharmacology* 45, no. 5 (September–October 2013): 508–12, doi.org/10.4103/0253-7613.117784.

128 **magnesium (in the glycinate form):** S. B. Sartori et al., "Magnesium Deficiency Induces Anxiety and HPA Axis Dysregulation: Modulation by Therapeutic Drug Treatment," *Neuropharmacology* 62, no. 1 (January 2012): 304–12, doi.org/10.1016/j.neuropharm.2011.07.027.

134 **decimate the beneficial bacteria:** Aparna Shil and Havovi Chichger, "Artificial Sweeteners Negatively Regulate Pathogenic Characteristics of Two Model Gut Bacteria, *E. coli* and *E. faecalis*," *International Journal of Molecular Sciences* 22, no. 10 (May 15, 2021): 5228, doi.org/10.3390/ijms22105228.

136 **foods rich in magnesium:** J. F. Lu and C. H. Nightingale, "Magnesium Sulfate in Eclampsia and Pre-eclampsia: Pharmacokinetic Principles," *Clinical Pharmacokinets* 38, no. 4 (April 2000): 305–14, doi.org/10.2165/00003088-200038040-00002.

136 **potassium-rich foods:** Tommaso Filippini et al., "Potassium Intake and Blood Pressure: A Dose-Response Meta-Analysis of Randomized Controlled Trials," *Journal of the American Heart Association* 9, no. 12 (June 5, 2020): e015719, doi.org/10.1161/JAHA.119.015719.

136 **poor calcium metabolism:** I. C. Udenze et al., "Calcium and Magnesium Metabolism in Pre-Eclampsia," *West African Journal of Medicine* 33, no. 3 (July–September 2014): 178–82, PMID: 26070821.

136 **don't eat enough protein:** Punyatoya Bej et al., "Determination of Risk Factors for Pre-eclampsia and Eclampsia in a Tertiary Hospital of India: A Case Control Study," *Journal of Family Medicine and Primary Care* 2, no. 4 (October–December 2013): 371–75, doi.org/10.4103/2249-4863.123924.

Chapter 7: Nutritional Needs and Third Trimester Changes

142 **full twenty grams more:** Mary M. Murphy et al., "Adequacy and Sources of Protein Intake among Pregnant Women in the United States, NHANES 2003-2012," *Nutrients* 13, no. 3 (February 28, 2021): 795, doi.org/10.3390/nu13030795.

144 **reduce the chance of developing preeclampsia:** Mahsa Nordqvist, et al., "Timing of Probiotic Milk Consumption during Pregnancy and Effects on the Incidence of Preeclampsia and Preterm Delivery: A Prospective Observational Cohort Study in Norway," *BMJ Open* 8, no. 1 (January 2018): e018021, doi.org/10.1136/bmjopen-2017-018021.

Chapter 8: Preparing for the Big Day

151 **delay cord clamping:** Nisha Rana et al., "Effect of Delayed Cord Clamping of Term Babies on Neurodevelopment at 12 Months: A Randomized Controlled Trial," *Neonatology* 115, no. 1 (2019): 36–42, doi.org/10.1159/000491994.

152 **twenty-four hours before bathing:** Susan Warren et al., "Effects of Delayed Newborn Bathing on Breastfeeding, Hypothermia, and Hypoglycemia." *Journal for Obstetrics, Gynecologic, and Neonatal Nursing* 49, no. 2 (March 2020): 181–89, doi.org/10.1016/j.jogn.2019.12.004.

152 **shorten the second stage of labor:** Michele Simpson et al., "Raspberry Leaf in Pregnancy: Its Safety and Efficacy in Labor," *Journal of Midwifery & Women's Health* 46, no. 2 (March–April 2001): 51–59, doi.org/10.1016/s1526-9523(01)00095-2.

153 **six dates a day:** O. Al-Kuran et al., "The Effect of Late Pregnancy Consumption of Date Fruit on Labour and Delivery," *Journal of Obstetrics and Gynaecology* 3, no. 1 (January 31, 2011): 29–31, doi.org/10.3109/01443615.2010.522267.

CHAPTER 9: FOODS FOR RECOVERY

166 **postpartum women experience thyroiditis:** Sara Naji Rad and Linda Deluxe, "Postpartum Thyroiditis," *StatPearls*, updated June 21, 2022, PMID: 32491578, ncbi.nlm.nih.gov/books/NBK557646/.

167 **need an extra 670 calories:** K. Dewey, "Energy and Protein Requirements during Lactation," *Annual Review of Nutrition* 17 (1997): 19–36, doi.org/10.1146/annurev.nutr.17.1.19.

169 **causes of postpartum depression:** Yu-Hung Lin et al., "Association between Postpartum Nutritional Status and Postpartum Depression Symptoms," *Nutrients* 11, no. 6 (May 28, 2019): 1204, doi.org/10.3390/nu11061204.

170 **reduce PPD by as much as 50 percent:** Leda Chatzi et al., "Dietary Patterns during Pregnancy and the Risk of Postpartum Depression: The Mother-Child 'Rhea' Cohort in Crete, Greece," *Public Health Nutrition* 14, no. 9 (September 14, 2011): 1663–70, doi.org/10.1017/S1368980010003629.

CHAPTER 10: NUTRITION FOR NURSING

176 **at three months of age:** Iná S. Santos, Alicia Matijasevich, and Marlos R. Domingues; "Maternal Caffeine Consumption and Infant Nighttime Waking: Prospective Cohort Study," *Pediatrics* 129, no. 5 (May 2012): 860–68, doi.org/10.1542/peds.2011-1773.

177 **5 to 6 percent of what the mother drinks:** Julie Mennella, "Alcohol's Effect on Lactation," *Alcohol Research & Health* 25, no. 3 (2001): 230–34, https://www.ncbi.nlm.nih.gov/pmc/articles/PMC6707164.

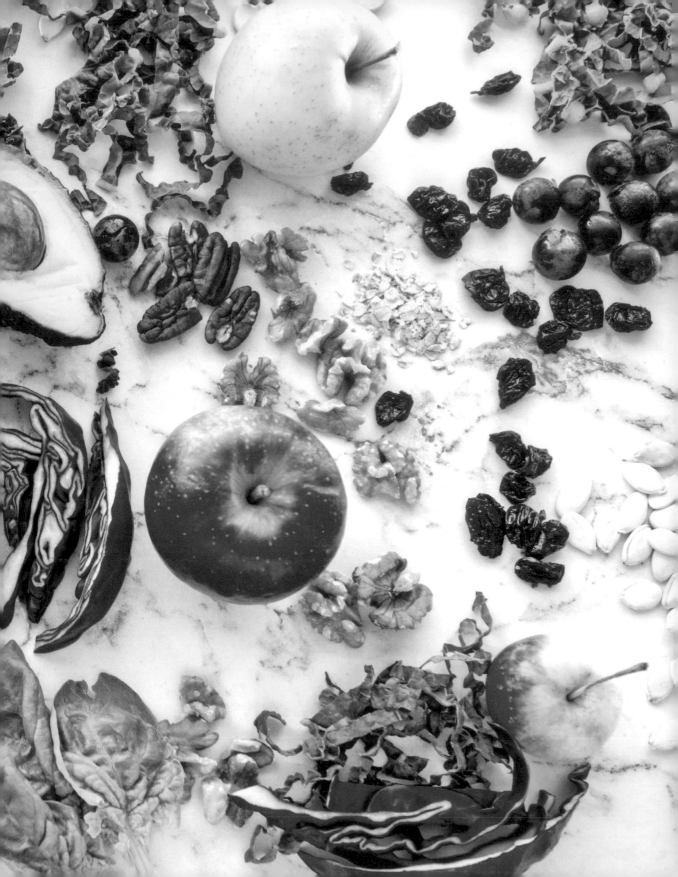

INDEX

Note: Italicized page numbers indicate material in tables or illustrations.

Ginger Veggie Fried Rice, 211–14
glucose, 103, 130
glycine, 167
grains, 57, 81, 91, 111
Granola Bars, Homemade, 203–5
grapes, 60
grass-fed meats, 58, 59
green beans, 60
Green Smoothie, 191–92
green tea, 71
green vegetables, 51, 54, 70, 124
grocery delivery, 149

hair loss, 165
HALT strategy, 109, 180
headaches, 63, 129
heartbeat, rapid or palpitations, 23
hemoglobin A1c, 24–25, 133
hempseed protein powder, 82
herbs, 62, 85
high blood pressure, 135
Homemade Granola Bars, 203–5
honey, 86, 155
honeydew melon, 60
hormones
    and dietary fats, 51
    in first trimester, 12–13
    and hair loss, 165
    monitoring, 166
    and morning sickness, 64
    and nesting period, 148
    postpartum, 163, 165, 167
    in third trimester, 148
hot peppers, 60
human chorionic gonadotropin (hCG), 13, 64
hunger, 45, 102, 103, 109, 115, 174

immune system, 73, 88, 167, 171–72
insomnia, 128
insulin, 130
insurance, 23, 25
iodine, *20, 34*, 40, 41, *122*, 142, 168
iron, *20*, 37–38
    and anemia, 167
    boosting intake of, 42
    and constipation, 68
    deficiency in, 23, 42, 167
    heme and nonheme, 20, 40–41, 144

from organ meats, 48
and postpartum depression, 170
and postpartum recovery, 166, 167
and supplements, *34*, 144
testing, 22, 23, 166
in third trimester, 143–44
and vegetarians/vegans, 22, 40–41
irritable bowel syndrome (IBS), 91

jumping while pregnant, 123

kale, 60
kefir, 91, 144, 168
kimchi, 54, 91, 144
kiwis, 60
kombucha, 79

labor, foods to induce, 152–53
Labor-Ade, recipe for, 156
labor and birth
    bleeding after, 163, 164
    and delaying clamping umbilical
        cord, 151
    and delaying washing baby, 151–52
    emotional responses to, 157
    first days and weeks after, 163–65
    foods/beverages for active labor, 154–56
    foods/beverages for after delivery, 156–57
    foods to induce labor, 152–53
    and placenta, 151
    recovering from birth, 147–48
    soreness following, 164
lactation classes and consultants,
    150–51, 172
Lactobacillus acidophilus, 39
Lactobacillus rhamnosus, 39
lactogenic foods, 175, 257–66
lactose intolerance, 50
La Leche League, 172
laxatives, 164
leafy green vegetables, 41, 68, 70, 124, 164
leftovers, 111
leg cramps, 63, 127
legumes, 47, 81, 91, 143
Lemon-Coconut Energy Bites, 261–62
Lemon Sole with Fried Capers, 241–42